The POISONING of OUR CHILDREN

Fighting the Obesity Epidemic in America

By Keeley C. Drotz, RD

Foreword by Don R. Russell, DO, MS, FAAP

TGBG NUTRITION PUBLISHING

MCKINNEY, TEXAS

The Poisoning of Our Children
Fighting the Obesity Epidemic in America

This title is also available as an ebook.
Visit PoisoningOurChildren.com

Cover and Book Design by Drotz Design

Published by:
TGBG Nutrition Publishing
McKinney, Texas
TGBGnutrition.com

Printed in the United States of America

ISBN: 978-0-578-10524-6

Library of Congress Control Number: 2012939419

Dedication and Acknowledgments

Because the name of my business is TGBG Nutrition Counseling Services – "To God Be the Glory" – it only makes sense that, first and foremost, this book is dedicated to God. His truths inspired these pages and I could not have written this book without Him. God gets one hundred percent of the credit for this book, as well as for any of the good that results from it. I give you all of the glory, Lord.

Secondly, I want to thank my wonderful, loving husband, Dallas. Without his help, strong support and encouragement, listening ear, and even "prodding" at times, this book would have never been started, not to mention finished. Whether this book sells one or one million copies, Dallas is my biggest fan and would have insisted that I write it, no matter what. He is also solely responsible for the book design. Thank you, baby – I love you with all of my heart.

I also want to thank my sweet, beautiful daughters, Nevaya and Adelyn, who have taught me so much more than I ever learned from books. They have truly been an inspiration for this book, and much that I have learned through their precious lives is contained in these pages. You girls are my greatest joy.

I am forever grateful and deeply indebted to my mom and dad for raising me and my sister in a loving Christian home, as well as encouraging and enabling me to pursue a career in the field of nutrition. Thank you for everything. I love you both very much.

This book would not have made it to publication without my brilliant editor, Kathy Altaras. Thank you for being exceedingly patient and flexible with me. You are amazing to work with and I sincerely appreciate all of your help.

Lastly, thank you to all of the clients and families that I have worked with over the years – without my encounters and experiences with you, I would have nothing to write. You have taught me more than I ever learned in school.

MEDICAL DISCLAIMER

The information contained in this book is intended to complement, not substitute for, the advice of your child's pediatrician. Do not rely on the information in this book as an alternative to medical advice from your child's pediatrician. Before starting any dietary or physical activity program, consult with your child's pediatrician. He or she can discuss your child's individual needs and provide appropriate counseling and guidance. If you have questions regarding how the information in this book applies to your child, speak to your child's pediatrician. Never delay seeking medical advice, disregard medical advice, or discontinue medical treatment because of information contained in this book.

CONTENTS

Foreword

Our children are going to die younger than we will. The average life span of our children's generation, and our grandchildren's generation, will be shorter than the average life span of our generation. Think about this, for the very first time in the history of mankind, the next generation will not live as long as their parents! In the time of Jesus and Caesar Augustus, the average life span of a Roman citizen was approximately thirty-five years. Today, the average life span of a U.S. citizen is more than seventy-five years. What has caused this dramatic increase in human life, such that the potential for human longevity is over twice as long as it was at the peak of the Roman Empire? It has been the vast improvements in sanitation, medical knowledge and care, living conditions, transportation, and nutrition that have allowed successive generations to live longer. This has been especially true in the last two hundred years.

So then, why is it that our children and our grandchildren may not live as long as us? Have we seen a sudden decrease in sanitation? Has medical knowledge and care disappeared? Have our living conditions or transportation capabilities horribly changed? Obviously, these are not the answers. Ironically, this dramatic change in longevity is occurring because of a veritable cornucopia of food and food choices. Over the last several generations we have seen marked improvements in the ability to feed our population, but now those very same life-changing benefits are turning on us and becoming life-threatening challenges. Instead of having insufficient access to food, we have an overabundance of available food, a vast array of both good and bad food choices and a cacophony of ways our food is being processed. Combine this with a more sedentary lifestyle and we have created an environment where our children are becoming obese, which leads to an increased risk of high cholesterol, high blood pressure, diabetes, and liver disease. Altogether, this makes up what is known as the Metabolic Syndrome. This, in turn, may result in the untimely and early deaths of our children and our grandchildren.

Infants and children up to the age of two or three have a natural ability to sense when they are full and they will automatically stop eating. We actually have to teach our children how to overeat and make bad nutritional choices. They learn these bad habits from television ads and other media, they learn them from the meals they receive at school, but mostly our children learn poor nutritional habits from their parent's lifestyles. It is easier to stop and get "fast-food" or pop prepared and processed foods into the microwave instead of taking the extra time to prepare a more nutritious home-cooked meal. When we adopt these "easier" lifestyle choices, we may be shortening our children's lives. The results of our actions may not be seen for decades, but the poison seed has already been planted in childhood.

Keeley Drotz has written a marvelous book, easy to read and full of practical information on how to keep our children healthier and happier. As a mother, she has presented practical suggestions that other care providers can follow. As a pediatrician, I have found many things in her book that I have incorporated into my daily practice. Keeley's book will allow us to be better parents.

Don R. Russell, DO, MS, FAAP
Evergreen Children's Clinic
Puyallup, Washington

Preface

When I initially decided to pursue a career in nutrition, I was disheartened to learn that I would be referred to as a "Registered Dietitian." I did not want the word, or more importantly, the connotation of the word "diet" as part of my lifelong professional title. To an adolescent female, the term "diet" holds negative implications. I had been on diets, most of my friends had been on diets, many family members had been on diets – all of them failed. Thus, I did not like the word and was adamantly opposed to being associated with it.

"Diet"

According to the *American Heritage Dictionary*, the word "diet" (as a noun) means, "the usual food and drink of a person," or, "something used, enjoyed, or provided regularly."[1] But the term "diet" as Americans typically refer to it is the verb form: "I am dieting," or, "I am going to diet," which means, "to eat and drink according to a regulated system, especially so as to lose weight or control a medical condition."[2]

The thesaurus gives synonyms for the verb "diet," which include: "abstain," "starve," "fast," "slenderize," "cut down," "cut back," and "reduce."[3] These are the connotations that the word "diet" conveys to the average American. I preferred not to have any of these terms attached to myself in any way, most especially "starve." Not exactly a boost to my career. But after hours and hours of research, it was very clear that the only way to be a college-educated, professional, credible, and credentialed "nutritionist" was, in fact, to become a "registered *diet*itian."

"Nutrition"

*Nutrition*ist – that sounded much more appropriate, noble, distinguished. The *American Heritage Dictionary* states that the word "nutrition" means, "the process of nourishing or being nourished, especially the process by which a living organism assimilates food and uses it for growth and for replacement of tissues."[4] I liked that – that is what I desired to study and be associated with.

Synonyms for "nutrition" listed in the thesaurus are: "nourishment," "sustenance," and "food."[5] I equate nutrition with health, well-being, vibrancy. But as it turns out, nearly anyone can hang up a shingle and call themselves a "nutritionist." Sure, he or she may have taken a six-week course and have a certificate of some kind, but they are not credible nor are they acknowledged by the medical community.

So, in the end, I resolved this issue by referring to myself as a dietitian/nutritionist. I learned in my early years of practice that this is what most other dietitians do as well; we are basically forced to do so. If I tell someone that I am a "dietitian" for a living, they give me a look that says, "You are a what?" And I end up saying, "I am a nutritionist," anyway. Or they assume I am confined to a hospital basement writing menus and preparing institutional food (which my grandmother still thinks I do). As a result, I now skip the very confused facial expressions and incorrect assumptions and just answer the question, "What do you do?" with, "I am a dietitian/nutritionist." It solves the problem.

"Anti-Diet" Dietitian

My point is this: I am what I refer to as the "anti-diet" dietitian. If I could eliminate the word "diet" from my title, I would. But I am stuck with it. So I am "anti-diet." And it works. I have never put a single client or patient on a "diet" or told anyone to follow a "diet." In fact, I spend at least the first appointment with each patient explaining how to completely shift their thoughts about the term "diet." It is much like a deprogramming session because Americans have been programmed to believe that we need to follow a "diet" in order to lose weight. And it is having the opposite effect, causing weight gain – faster and in larger amounts than ever before. Yes, I give my patients meal plans and guidelines to follow – but the term "diet" is not in my vocabulary, nor are counting calories or fat grams. Guidance and parameters are offered as a way to help clients change habits and establish a healthy lifestyle, but there is no focus on a "diet" or restricting specific foods.

Therefore, in this book about combating and preventing obesity and chronic disease, there will not be any recommendations about following a particular diet or even starting a diet per se – so you can breathe a sigh of relief. However, if you were hoping to find lose-weight-quick diet or exercise recommendations, I apologize. If you are not yet convinced that quick-fix fad diets and exercise regimens do not work for permanent weight loss and maintenance, or for reducing the risk of chronic disease, I hope that this book persuades you to believe otherwise.

The Obesity Epidemic in America

I wrote this book because, after counseling numerous patients of all ages, genders, and ethnicities, I started asking myself, 'Why have overweight and poor health among children and adults become such an issue in our country in recent years? And why were they not significant issues in the past? What has changed so dramatically over the past twenty, thirty, forty years to make it not only a problem or concern, but the epidemic that it is today?' And I started to see a trend, both in my professional work and in my day-to-day life as a wife, mother, daughter, and friend. I observed the same core issues again and again, and arrived at some preliminary conclusions regarding the epidemic of overweight and obesity in America. And that is when I began to more thoroughly research the existing studies and data on the topic, which are referenced throughout this book.

One of my areas of specialization is providing nutrition counseling and education to overweight children, adolescents, and their families. This experience, coupled with my research, helped pinpoint some of the major contributors – and solutions – to overweight and obesity, particularly among children and adolescents. At the same time, I was writing articles pertaining to childhood nutrition for a website, HealthCastle.com. While I enjoyed composing the articles, I grew discouraged because I was unable to adequately address the issue of childhood obesity in the space allowed by a single article.

Around that time, a friend of mine that worked as a dietitian at a weight management center made a statement that ultimately convinced me to write this book. She said that the obesity epidemic puts dietitians to shame. I pondered her words and realized, 'You know, she is right! Here I am, specifically educated, trained, and prepared to go out and combat the problem of overweight and obesity, yet the health of our nation only grows worse. What does that imply? I am not doing my job!' So I wrote this book with the desire fulfill my role as a dietitian to the best of my ability: To make Americans aware of the severity of childhood obesity and the likelihood that it will result in chronic disease, to explain the factors that have led to the epidemic of childhood obesity in America today, and finally, to offer practical solutions to prevent and treat this condition.

1 THE POISONING OF OUR CHILDREN

A humbling reality is that the daily habits that have become pervasive in modern-day America are poisoning the bodies and minds of children and adolescents. Would parents inject their offspring with a chemical that causes disease? "No way," you answer, "are you completely crazy?!" Yet parents regularly allow children to consume soda, sweetened beverages, candy, chips, fast-food, and meals out of a can, box, freezer, or microwave. As if that is not enough, they let them stay inside and watch television or play video games rather than go outside and play. Parents are, in effect, poisoning children each time they permit these activities. They may as well give kids a shot that causes obesity, diabetes, heart disease, and cancer, among a host of other ailments, because it is projected that children born today will live shorter, sicklier lives than their parents and grandparents. And it is solely related to the American lifestyle. Not only are children's bodies being affected, so are their minds. By allowing – even enabling – youths to establish unhealthy habits early on, adults are conveying that these behaviors and mindsets are acceptable. These toxic beliefs seep into every part of their being until kids are unable to recognize what is healthy as opposed to unhealthy, what is beneficial compared to what is damaging, and what might cause them to become sick versus that which will strengthen their bodies and fight disease. Youngsters do not know any differently; they are unaware that there is a way to improve their quality of life.

A main objective of this book is the prevention and reversal of obesity and chronic disease among children and adolescents, as these are pivotal periods for addressing weight issues and health conditions. This is partly because infancy, the preschool years, and adolescence/puberty are critical stages of growth and development which involve the formation and development of fat cells.[1,2] It is also more effective to prevent or treat weight and medical problems in a youngster than in an adult. Obesity is rather challenging and expensive to treat once it occurs, and after an individual becomes significantly overweight, it is particularly difficult to achieve and maintain a healthy body weight.[3] This does not even take into consideration the health consequences that may develop in the meantime. As a result, the prevention of obesity altogether is the most effective strategy for combating this epidemic. Nevertheless, many of the recommendations in this book are applicable to adults as well.

While most Americans are cognizant of concerns pertaining to childhood and adolescent obesity, few seem to realize the magnitude of the problem. First of all, obesity among American youth has become a leading public health concern, which means it now sits atop a list with such medical conditions as heart disease and cancer.[4] Consequently, the prevention of obesity among children and adolescents has become a health priority in this country.[5] To further convey the severity of the issue, this chapter will provide detailed background information regarding childhood and adolescent obesity and chronic disease. In addition, each subsequent chapter contains facts and statistics for the purpose of convincing readers that childhood obesity is not only a real problem, but that there are proven contributing factors. As such, there are specific lifestyle and dietary modifications that can aid in preventing and reversing the continued spread of this epidemic.

I am well aware that some readers may disagree with certain conclusions that are drawn in this book, and this is to be expected. Every individual is entitled to his or her own opinions and beliefs. The goal of this book is not to be "right" or purport that I have all the answers. The purpose of these pages is to present American citizens with sound evidence based upon the findings of credible research studies coupled with my experiences and observations as a dietitian working with children and their families. My hope and desire is that families find even one or two changes that they can initially adopt rather seamlessly, and then over time, possibly adjust to another modification or two. Adopting healthier habits does not have to be accomplished all at once. But gradually, the American lifestyle can begin to reflect health and wellness.

The Definitions of Overweight and Obesity

For the purposes of this book, it is unnecessary to clearly define and differentiate between the clinical terms of overweight and obesity, as this can be quite complicated, especially when discussing children and adolescents. Do note, however, that the clinical definitions of overweight and obesity are utilized in reference to statistics and studies. For the entirety of this book, although the clinical definitions underlie the terms, it is acceptable to think of overweight as an individual who weighs more than he should (because of excess body fat) based on height, and obesity as someone who weighs considerably more than she ought to (due to excess body fat) based on height.

Familiarity with the term "Body Mass Index," otherwise known as BMI, is important because it is used throughout this book and is terminology with which all Americans should be comfortable. It will also help clarify the clinical cut-off points for overweight and obesity. BMI is now widely accepted as a reliable and valid measurement of weight status among all age groups and is routinely used for this purpose.[6] Body mass index is essentially the comparison of a person's weight to his or her height. Technically, BMI is calculated as: weight in kilograms divided by the square of the height in meters (weight in kilograms/height in meters^2). There is also a formula to calculate BMI using weight in pounds and height in inches. Although it has its limitations, and no method is perfect, studies have shown that BMI does correlate well with total body fat in most individuals.[7] It is important to recognize that BMI does not measure body fat directly; as a result, some individuals – such as athletes – may have a higher body mass index (because of muscle mass) that classifies them as overweight even though they have no excess body fat. Conversely, those who have lost muscle mass, such as the elderly, may also obtain inaccurate BMI results.

The use of body mass index is rather straightforward among adults: weight status is classified according to the number that is derived from the BMI equation (which becomes known as the individual's "BMI"; refer to Table 1). Among children and adolescents, the application of BMI is not as simple. A "normal" and healthy amount of body fat – and thus a "normal" and healthy BMI – varies dramatically during the early years. This is because as children and adolescents grow and develop, the degree of body fat that is normal varies with each age and stage (and gender). Thus, BMI percentiles have been developed for children and adolescents which are gender- and age-specific. After a child's BMI has been calculated, it is plotted on a gender-specific BMI-for-age growth chart (see Figure 1). This shows which percentile the child's BMI falls within, and it is this percentile that reveals whether a child or adolescent is underweight, within the healthy range, overweight/ at-risk of obesity, or obese (refer to Table 2).

Table 1: Body Mass Index Classification: Adults[8,9]

BMI (kg/m^2)	Weight Classification
Less than 18.5	Underweight
18.5 - 24.9	Normal (Healthy) Weight
25.0 - 29.9	Overweight (Pre-Obese)
30 - 34.9	Obesity Class 1
35 - 39.9	Obesity Class 2 (Moderate Obesity)
Equal to or Greater than 40	Obesity Class 3 (Extreme/Morbid Obesity)

Figure 1: Growth Chart[10]

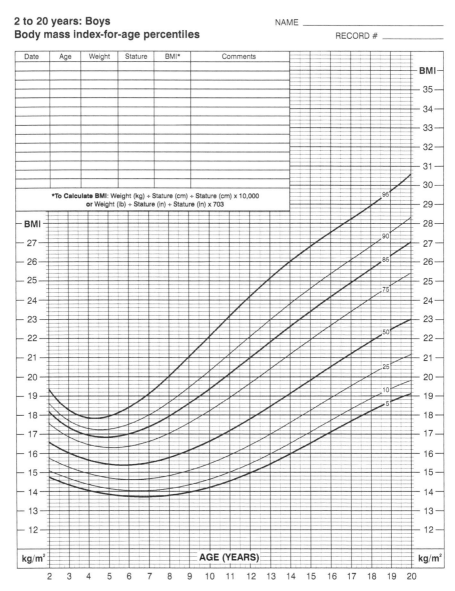

2 to 20 years: Boys
Body mass index-for-age percentiles

NAME _____

RECORD # _____

Published May 30, 2000 (modified 10/16/00).
SOURCE: Developed by the National Center for Health Statistics in collaboration with
the National Center for Chronic Disease Prevention and Health Promotion (2000).
http://www.cdc.gov/growthcharts

SAFER · HEALTHIER · PEOPLE™

Table 2: Body Mass Index Percentile Classification: Children and Adolescents[11]

BMI Percentile	Weight Classification
Less than the 5th	Underweight
5th to Less than the 85th	Healthy Weight
85th to Less than 95th	Overweight (At risk of Obesity)
Equal to or Greater than the 95th	Obese

The Increase in Overweight and Obesity

After remaining relatively stable during the 1960s and 1970s, rates of overweight and obesity in the United States have escalated so dramatically that it is now considered to be an epidemic.[12,13] Overweight and obesity are not limited to a single population group: increases have occurred in both genders, as well as all age levels and ethnic groups.[14] Despite numerous advances in medicine and public health, a greater number of Americans than ever carry excess weight, and the number of overweight children and adolescents has reached an alarming rate.

At least two-thirds of adults in the United States are overweight or obese; contrast that with the late 1970s, when less than half of the adult population was classified as such.[15,16] Obesity alone (notice that is *obesity*, not simply overweight) climbed from an estimated fifteen percent in the late 1970s to over thirty-four percent today; in other words, obesity prevalence increased by more than two-fold during the past thirty years.[17] Even worse, extreme obesity has multiplied greater than four times.

Children and Adolescents

Astonishingly, a diagnosis of overweight is now the most prevalent medical condition among children in the United States.[18] Furthermore, America is a leading nation in terms of overweight and obese youth, second only to Malta.[19] While research shows that obesity tends to be particularly high among Black, Hispanic, and low-income populations, this book addresses American youth as a whole because obesity has become more prevalent in every group, and health and wellness is important for all children.

The most recent statistics reveal that approximately seventeen percent of children between the ages of two and nineteen in this country are classified as obese (note: that is *obese*, not simply overweight).[20] Over the course of a few decades, the number of obese preschoolers two to five years old doubled; the percentage of obese school-aged children between six and eleven years old tripled; and the proportion of obese adolescent twelve to nineteen year olds nearly quadrupled (please refer to Figure 2).[21] These numbers do not include those that are overweight/at-risk of becoming obese, which includes a significant of proportion children and adolescents.

Figure 2: Obesity Trends for Children/Adolescents in the U.S., 1963-2008[22]

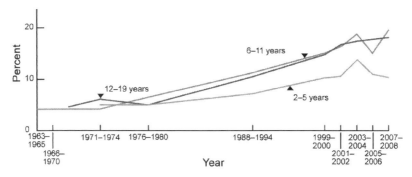

The Consequences of Overweight and Obesity

If the trend towards overweight and obesity remains at the current level – and it shows no signs of reversing – it will have a detrimental impact on future generations. The consequences are appalling: Obesity, largely related to poor diet and inadequate physical activity, is a major cause of preventable disease and death in the United States.[23] It is well-established that obesity leads to early death.[24,25] Compared with individuals of a healthy weight, those who are obese have a significantly higher risk of death from all causes, especially cardiovascular conditions.[26,27] Approximately 145 to 185 thousand deaths per year in this country are related to overweight and obesity.[28] Interpreted another way, an unhealthy diet and lack of physical activity are associated with as many as 145 to 185 thousand deaths in the United States every year.

Among adults, overweight and obesity are known to increase the risk of cardiovascular disease, type 2 diabetes, elevated cholesterol and triglyceride levels, high blood pressure, stroke, cancer, sleep apnea, asthma and other respiratory problems, arthritis, gallbladder disease, surgical complications, and a host of other physical and health problems.[29,30] In females, obesity is associated with a higher incidence of menstrual irregularities and fertility problems, as well as complications of pregnancy.[31] Excess weight can make existing chronic conditions even worse. Moreover, overweight and obese adults often experience discrimination and stigmatization, as well as suffer from a poor body image.

Children and Adolescents

Over the last thirty years, adults have remained silent observers
as weight problems among children and adolescents have become
widespread, assuming that there are no adverse effects until
adulthood. Health professionals and parents alike used to believe that
eating healthfully and exercising were important for adults, but not
as much for children. To their dismay, it is now evident that there are
severe and immediate consequences of excess weight among youth.

As a matter of fact, medical problems are actually quite
common among obese children and adolescents: they are at
high risk for type 2 diabetes, insulin resistance/impaired glucose
tolerance, elevated cholesterol and triglyceride levels, high blood
pressure, asthma, sleep apnea, gastrointestinal and liver issues,
early maturation, menstrual irregularities/polycystic ovarian
syndrome, and foot and other orthopedic problems, among other
health issues (refer to Figure 3).[32,33] Overweight youngsters are
more likely to be diagnosed with at least one, if not several, risk
factors for cardiovascular disease, leading to a greater chance that
they will experience heart and/or vascular disease in adulthood,
if not before.[34] Type 2 diabetes, a disease once limited to the adult
population (in fact, it was once referred to as adult-onset diabetes),
is now on the rise among children and adolescents – something
the medical community never imagined possible. This has been
attributed to the increased incidence of overweight and obesity
in this population.[35] Additionally, overweight and obese children
and adolescents are much more likely to be overweight or obese
as adults.[36,37] For instance, approximately one out of every three

obese preschoolers and one in two obese school-aged children will be obese as an adult.[38] Furthermore, medical problems related to childhood and adolescent obesity tend to persist into adulthood.[39,40]

Oftentimes, overweight children and adolescents experience social and psychological issues such as stigmatization, depression, poor self-image, low self-esteem, extreme dieting, and eating disorders – especially during adolescence.[41,42] The young people I counsel regarding weight issues usually suffer from very poor self-esteem, which is devastating at such a critical stage of their lives. It is disheartening to say the least, because matters of self-worth are inherent during childhood and adolescence, regardless of weight issues.

There is more: it is believed that the epidemic of childhood and adolescent obesity in the United States will result in a decreased life expectancy for future generations.[43] For the first time in decades, Americans have to face the reality that their children and grandchildren may very well live shorter lives than they will.

Although beyond the scope of this book, the economic impact of obesity in this country is staggering. The money that is being spent is unnecessary, because obesity and its associated health conditions are entirely preventable. Furthermore, the billions invested into research on curing these preventable diseases, such as type 2 diabetes and cardiovascular disease, could be saved by addressing the lifestyle factors that contribute to the development of these conditions in the first place – and doing so early on, during childhood. Simply stated, by implementing lifestyle changes, Americans can save themselves and other Americans billions and billions of dollars each year.

Figure 3: Complications of Childhood and Adolescent Obesity

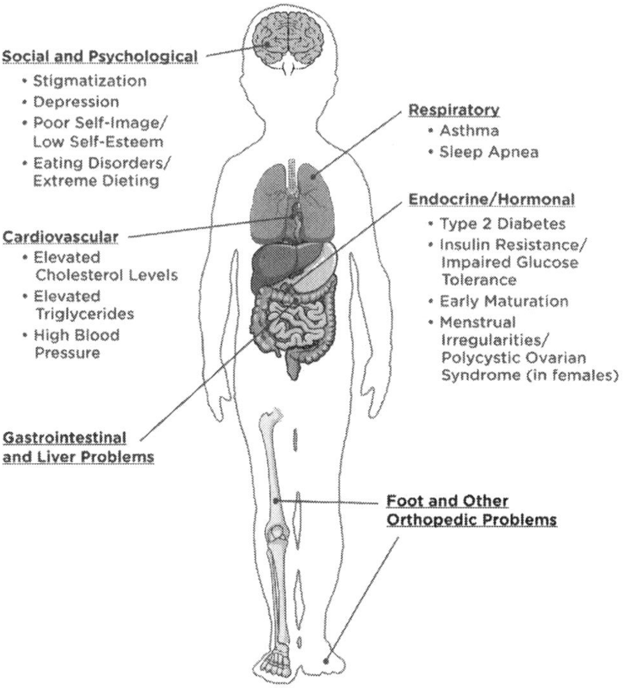

Social and Psychological
- Stigmatization
- Depression
- Poor Self-Image/
  Low Self-Esteem
- Eating Disorders/
  Extreme Dieting

Respiratory
- Asthma
- Sleep Apnea

Endocrine/Hormonal
- Type 2 Diabetes
- Insulin Resistance/
  Impaired Glucose
  Tolerance
- Early Maturation
- Menstrual
  Irregularities/
  Polycystic Ovarian
  Syndrome (in females)

Cardiovascular
- Elevated
  Cholesterol Levels
- Elevated
  Triglycerides
- High Blood
  Pressure

**Gastrointestinal
and Liver Problems**

**Foot and Other
Orthopedic Problems**

Gastric Bypass and Weight Reduction Surgery

Gastric bypass and other weight-reduction surgeries are currently being performed at an all-time high. Instead of diligently working to prevent the unwanted problem of obesity, Americans now have the option of undergoing a "simple" procedure to become rid of it. The trouble with this type of thinking is that the patient does not realize how invasive the procedure is (on many levels: physical, emotional, financial, and so on) – nor the complications that may result – until after the surgery has been performed. The mentality in America is in danger of becoming, "I am overweight, but that is all right. I can still eat this candy bar even though I am not really hungry, and watch

TV rather than go outside and be active. After all, I can have gastric bypass surgery someday." Although this may sound far-fetched, it is the road this nation is headed down. Even if they do not reach this extreme, many Americans have come to rely upon prescription medications – a handful of pills – to combat a host of chronic conditions, such as high cholesterol and high blood pressure, which are related to an unhealthy weight and lifestyle.

The truth is that there are some severely obese individuals who are unable to lose weight despite how hard they may try, and in these cases, gastric bypass or another weight reduction surgery might be an option to consider. However, this should be the exception – not routine as it has become. Many state medical insurance plans reimburse for gastric bypass surgery, which is an expensive procedure. This means that taxpayers are paying for these patients to undergo weight reduction surgery. While such surgeries have helped those who could not have achieved weight loss by any other means, a more positive and proactive approach is to direct that money towards the prevention of obesity to begin with: to programs in schools, to parent education classes in the community, and to medical and public-health institutions aimed at addressing and reversing this crisis. A purpose of this book is to prevent gastric bypass and weight reduction surgeries from ever needing to be considered in the first place.

The Causes of Overweight and Obesity

There is no single cause of overweight or obesity. A person's weight is affected by multiple factors: genetic, metabolic, biological, psychological, behavioral, environmental, cultural, and socioeconomic.[44,45]

Although genetics do contribute to the development of overweight and obesity, heredity alone does not account for the rapid and significant increase that has occurred among all age groups during the last few decades.[46,47] Thus, it may be argued that behavioral and environmental influences are major causes of excessive weight gain.[48]

While there are many factors, this book will specifically examine the roles of diet, physical activity, and lifestyle in the obesity epidemic. Overweight and obesity are essentially the result of consistently eating more calories than one can burn off through physical activity; most cases of overweight and obesity result from the consumption of too many calories coupled with inadequate physical activity.[49,50] This is true for one hundred percent of the patients I counsel regarding weight issues. When an individual begins to eat healthier and be physically active on a regular basis, he or she immediately loses a significant amount of weight and becomes healthier (based on laboratory data), regardless of the degree of obesity.

Examining behavioral and environmental changes that have occurred in American society over the past few decades, two major influences stand out related to diet, exercise, and lifestyle: an increased availability of high-calorie foods, which taste good and are often quick and easy grab, and a decrease in physical activity, including less active jobs, hobbies, and leisure-time pursuits.[51] Moreover, inordinate amounts of time spent on sedentary activities, such as watching television or playing video games, have grown especially prevalent and harmful among children and adolescents. These are just a few examples of modern-day habits that have resulted in increased rates of overweight and obesity in America. Human beings might not be able to alter their genes, but can – and desperately need to – adjust their thinking, behavior, and environment, especially in regards to dietary intake, physical activity levels, and lifestyle habits.

Weight Loss is Not the Main Focus

One point requires emphasis: the focus for every individual – and even the goal – is to strive to become healthier by developing positive habits. The goal is not necessarily to get down to an "ideal body weight." It is all about feeling better, improving overall well-being, and decreasing the likelihood of disease. Even modest weight loss can reduce the risk of chronic illness.[52] Of utmost importance is the promotion of health and wellness, regardless of weight status or medical condition. It is not about how you look or your appearance – being thin or slender – it is about being healthy and feeling good. Being "skinny," as America defines it, is not desirable or healthy anyway. Some people's body types are larger-boned or stockier, and that is perfectly fine. I have counseled children who will never be "thin" or even at a "healthy weight" based on the charts. They are just bigger kids, usually due to their genetics. However, they have become significantly overweight and unhealthy with elevated blood pressure, cholesterol, and triglycerides. Sometimes just losing (and keeping off) a modest amount of their excess weight – by being taught to eat healthier and be more active – enables them to become more fit and healthy. And they feel better about themselves. That is the goal. They might not achieve an "ideal" weight, but they are certainly at a more appropriate weight than they were before. More than that, they are healthy based on medical tests and they feel good. Equally important, they have developed healthy habits. And they will pass these beneficial habits on to others, including future generations.

Further, when weight becomes the main emphasis, children and teenagers become more susceptible to developing eating disorders, which is the exact opposite of the original intent. Although a thorough discussion of eating disorders falls outside the bounds of this book, please remember one thing as you read: always avoid focusing on weight or food. A balanced perspective is necessary when seeking to develop healthy habits – either extreme is extremely unhealthy.

In order to be safe, effective, and permanent, weight loss must be accomplished slowly and over time – whether the goal is to shed ten pounds or one hundred and ten pounds. And that is what the methods in this book will achieve – gradual, yet healthful and long-term, weight loss. Excess weight is not gained overnight, and it will not be lost overnight. But the short-term reward is feeling better, day-by-day. By the end of even just one month, there will be noticeable results from a changed lifestyle: your pants will not fit so tightly, you will have the ability to walk up the stairs without becoming winded, you will experience an improved mental outlook, and you will have more energy and be able to live life more fully.

The Battle Against Obesity Requires Transformation

The forthcoming changes prescribed in this book require complete lifestyle transformations. There are no impossible fad diets or exercise regimens recommended – in fact, there will not be a lot of mention about diet or exercise per se at all. It does not offer any quick-fixes because there are none; this is obvious because otherwise overweight, obesity, and chronic disease would not be on the rise as they are today. What this book does discuss is the necessity of altering mindsets, behaviors, and environments – lifestyles, and in a sense, culture – to make winning the battle against obesity and chronic disease not only a possibility, but a reality.

America boasts groundbreaking progress in modern medicine, yet preventable diseases continue to occur at startling rates; this is incomprehensible. It is ironic that obesity among both children and adults is spiraling out-of-control at a time when there are more fad diets than ever . . . more weight loss schemes . . . more books on the subject of weight loss, health, and fitness . . . more exercise regimens . . . more physical activity options . . . more diet pills . . . and more "lite" and low-fat foods than ever. Food manufacturers have formulated a plethora of low-calorie, non-fat, reduced-sugar, and even low-carbohydrate food and beverage products. Fitness gurus have devised extreme exercise routines designed to burn calories and fat, strengthen, and tone in record time. Yet overweight and obesity continue to skyrocket among all population groups. This clearly demonstrates that these methods are not addressing the root of the problem.

This book will reveal core issues underlying the obesity epidemic. Fighting this epidemic requires enormous commitment by each individual, by every family, and by entire communities. But as you have read, there are no other options. Either kids will live healthy, long, fulfilling lives – or they will suffer from myriad preventable diseases and conditions, live shorter lives than their parents and grandparents, and have poor self-images. Unless Americans institute dramatic changes, children in this nation will experience a severely impaired sense of well-being and quality of life.

The cause of the obesity epidemic is multi-factorial, thus the approach for preventing and reversing the problem must be as well. The following chapters will discuss ten major issues pervasive in American culture that have directly contributed to the rise of obesity and chronic disease among children and adolescents. In essence, this book calls for a cultural shift, a pendulum swing, a return to America's roots.

- Issue 1: "Breastfeeding is the Best Start" addresses the benefits of breastfeeding that are not being fully realized because of inadequate rates of breastfeeding in America.

- Issue 2: "Healthy Eating Habits Begin Early" establishes the fact that early habits are lifelong habits, and so parents must begin teaching children how to eat healthfully as early as infancy and toddlerhood.

- Issue 3: "A Healthy Breakfast" explains why it is critical to consume a nutritious morning meal, especially for children and adolescents, and how to make it a reality.

- Issue 4: "Wholesome Lunches and Snacks" addresses America's growing reliance on unhealthy, highly-processed convenience foods for lunches and snacks.

- Issues 5 and 6: "More Family Meals, Less Happy Meals®" demonstrates the necessity of eating out less often, as well as training children to plan and prepare balanced meals, regularly sitting down to nutritious family dinners, and modeling healthy eating patterns for children.

- Issue 7: "The Truth about Sweetened Beverages" describes the negative effects of sweetened beverages, their contribution to childhood obesity, and the importance of reducing consumption of these beverages.

- Issue 8: "Establishing Physical Activity Habits Early" emphasizes the need to begin instilling physical activity habits early on in children's lives. Because children begin developing habits early, being physically active is not only important for the immediate benefits, but for establishing it as a long-term lifestyle.

- Issue 9: "Too Much Screen Time" addresses the issue of American children and families spending excessive amounts of time in front of screen-containing technological devices (television, movies, video games, computers, smartphones, and tablets), which is a major contributor to the epidemic of overweight and obesity.

- Issue 10: "Healthy Sleep, Rest, and Relaxation Habits" focuses on the concern that today's families, children and adults alike, are overworked, overstressed, and overtired. The result is poor health – physical, mental, and spiritual.

The final chapter of this book, "A Byproduct of Our Culture," will uncover some of the root causes of these issues. But first, the next chapter will explain exactly who is responsible for preventing and treating obesity and chronic disease among American youth, and why this is the case.

2 FAMILY & PARENTAL RESPONSIBILITY

Peggy Frezon, author of Dieting with my Dog *(2011, Hubble &*
Hattie), shared her family's story in Guideposts Magazine. *Peggy*
felt the way that most parents do upon hearing that our child has a
health concern: shocked. At a routine physical, Peggy learned that
her eighteen year old son's cholesterol and triglyceride levels were
elevated, placing him at an increased risk for heart disease. In Peggy's
case, her son was not overweight; in fact, he was actively involved in
several sports. However, Peggy admits that Andy had never been a
healthy eater: "In the morning, he got going with fried eggs, stacks of
crisp bacon, and butter-slathered toast. He'd come home after games
wanting grilled cheese sandwiches, chicken nuggets, or pizza. The
only greens I'd seen him touch were cans of Mountain Dew. I blamed*
myself."[1] Peggy silently lamented, "Soon Andy would be in college.
How could I teach my son healthy eating in a few months when I
hadn't been able to in eighteen years?"

Back home, as she sorted through Andy's bag of baseball equipment,
Peggy prayed, "Lord, why did we equip him so well for baseball, but

not his health? I promise to try and teach him eat better. But help me!"
Gradually, Peggy was able to teach Andy to eat more nutritiously. She
started by making healthier, lower-fat versions of the foods he already
enjoyed. Today, Peggy happily reports that her son, now twenty-one
years old, will eat salad; although he doesn't necessarily enjoy it yet, he
is trying to, which is an enormous step in the right direction.

As illustrated by Peggy's story, it is imperative for parents and families
to accept responsibility for children's and adolescent's health. Both
Peggy and her husband immediately took ownership of Andy's health
and made significant changes in their lives. Thankfully Peggy and her
family have been successful, and through a change in his dietary habits,
Andy's cholesterol and triglyceride levels have begun to improve.

Parents Must Accept Responsibility

Ultimately, it is the responsibility of families and adults – namely
parents – to instill healthful behaviors in children. Parents are vitally
important in teaching and modeling healthy habits to our kids, and
this critical role is being recognized more and more.[2] As adults, we
are responsible for teaching and helping those in their formative
years, as well as being role models and setting positive examples
for them. But we are failing. Based on the current trajectory,
future generations will live shorter and more diseased lives than
their parents and grandparents.[3] If he so chooses, an adult can do
something about his weight; but a child, especially a young one, is
dependent upon an adult because he is unable to care for himself
on his own. We have enormous influence on our children's lives,
including the habits they will establish and maintain for a lifetime.

Thus, it is the duty of parents and other adult family members to provide children with a healthy foundation.

Parents are expected to nurture, love, teach, train, correct, and provide for our children. If we are obligated to do all these things, then we are also responsible for helping our kids maintain a healthy weight and stay well. Children are incapable of doing so on their own, and if parents neglect to train kids while they are young, they will be unable to do so as adults. While there are other adults involved in children's lives that help influence and mold them, in the end, the majority of responsibility for teaching and shaping appropriate behavior falls on the family; the primary focus must be on what occurs inside the home.

Meeting Children's Needs

Parents tend to put the needs of their children above our own almost one hundred percent of the time. In general, kids get attention when they need it, regardless of a parent's needs. This is especially true in urgent situations: no matter what else may be going on, if a child screams, we drop what we are doing and run to her. She receives full, undivided attention. It should be the same with issues of weight and health among our children – this, too, is a dire situation that requires us to put their needs before our own and give them complete, unwavering attention.

The health and well-being of our children is a need that we must help them meet; it is as just as vital as all of their other requirements. Parents are very effective at making sure our kids' needs are met, often going above and beyond, even if it means sacrificing in some way. Since we go the extra mile to make sure our children have the clothes, school items, and sporting equipment they need, as well as the toys, games, and gadgets they want, why not also ensure that they have the tools and habits required to live healthy, full lives? It is all too easy to be complacent in this area, but for the sake of our children, we need to make changes.

Shifting the Blame

Until they are able to do so for themselves, parents must take ownership of our children's lives and accept personal responsibility for their health. In order to do so, we have to stop shifting the blame. In America, it has become common to blame our genes for causing us to be overweight; blame our mother for not teaching us how to cook healthfully; blame the food industry for manufacturing delicious "fattening" foods; blame fast-food restaurants for serving artery-clogging hamburgers and fries; blame beverage companies for adding heaps of sugar to our favorite soda; blame television networks for producing entertaining programs that we like to sit and watch; and blame advertisement executives for successfully promoting unwholesome foods. On and on goes the blame game. American citizens have learned to rely on excuses over the past few decades. But the only way things are going to change for our children and our children's children is if someone stops making excuses. That someone needs to be us – the parents, guardians, caregivers, grandparents, and family members in children's lives.

The Foundation for Establishing Healthy Habits

First and foremost, the prevention and treatment of obesity and chronic disease must, absolutely must, begin in the home and with the family. There are no other options. In her book, *It's Never Too Soon to Discipline,* Dr. Ruth Peters states that, "Parents cannot look to educators, ministers, or pediatricians to teach their children responsibility and self-discipline."[4] She further clarifies herself, ". . . what some people lose sight of is that it is the parent's job to instill values, administer discipline, and serve as role models for their children."[5] These statements also apply to teaching and modeling healthy lifestyle habits.

Teachers are responsible for classrooms filled with twenty or more pupils, coaches oversee teams of no less than ten athletes, Sunday school teachers and youth group leaders are in charge of large numbers of students, and pediatricians see numerous patients each day. Due to sheer numbers, these leaders are simply unable to focus on every individual child. Moreover, instilling healthy habits and self-discipline are secondary concerns for these mentors because they have other primary objectives, such as teaching reading and math, training for athletics and sportsmanship, or providing medical care. In addition, parents spend greater amounts of time with our offspring than others do. Therefore, it is predominantly up to parents and adult family members to train and serve as examples for children about living healthy, whole lives. The aim of this book is to motivate and empower families to fulfill this role.

Parenting Style Adjustments

As Leslie Leyland Fields discusses in her article, *Five Myths of Parenting – Parent Traps,* it is a myth to believe that, "Good parenting produces happy children."[6] She goes on to explain that, "Many parents think the measurement of parenting is how happy the children are. If you are doing a good job, your child will be content. Toward this goal, you can engage in all kinds of questionable behavior. At least half of all American children have a TV in their bedrooms, for example, despite the growing evidence that it erodes health, study, and sleep habits. Many parents go into debt for their children, providing lavish birthday parties and exotic vacations. As obesity rates soar, parents fix the foods their children clamor for instead of what they need." Ms. Fields concludes her statements with the truth: "Trying to procure your child's happiness here and now is like catching river with a sieve. Do for your child what he cannot do for himself: distinguish between his short-term happiness and his long-term good."

Furthermore, Dr. Ruth Peters states in her book that, "Kids learn self-control when parents create boundaries and set limits."[7] According to the *American Heritage Dictionary*, self-control means: "control of one's emotions, desires, or actions by one's own will."[8] Alternative words for self-control include: self-discipline, willpower, restraint, strength of mind, strength of will, and self-will.[9] Therefore, parents need to create rules, boundaries, and limits in order for children to develop self-discipline, restraint, and willpower; in turn, this will enable them to establish healthy habits. Truthfully, these are traits that parents desire for children to develop anyway.

As families initiate lifestyle changes in an effort to teach children healthy habits and self-control, we will probably have to make some adjustments to our parenting styles. Because we prefer that our child not become an overweight sickly adult, we are going to have to say, "No," to the candy bar and, "Yes, you must go outside and play rather than watch television or play a video game." We must win the war against childhood obesity and disease, which means that initially, our children will probably be unhappy with us for setting boundaries. But after all, that is what being a parent is about. Eventually it will no longer be an issue because children will become accustomed to this new way of thinking, this changed behavior, and they will adopt healthy habits and self-discipline for themselves. And along the way, we help youngsters build character.

Dr. Peters admits that behavior modification can be challenging, but in the long-run, it is well worth it: "I'm not suggesting that this type of change is easy. Changing parenting styles can be quite tough. In fact, it can be downright awful! But even more disheartening is the realization later in your child's life that your adorable, overindulged little one has grown into a selfish, insecure, and unprepared adult. Do not lose focus on winning the battle (immediate kid satisfaction) while losing the war (adult happiness and self-respect). . . Think about it – it's never too soon to start setting limits, to say no to unreasonable requests, and to begin to build your child's character in a healthy way."[10] As she puts it so appropriately, "New things tend to frighten us, and fear is something we like to avoid. However, there are big stakes at risk here folks, and I think the payoff is worth the risk."[11] We must make changes for the sake of our children and our children's children, regardless of how frightened or intimidated we may feel. Their future – their very lives – are at stake.

Healthy Habits Must be Taught

In his book, *The New Dare to Discipline,* Dr. James Dobson states that, "Children also need to be taught *self*-discipline and responsible behavior. They need assistance in learning how to handle the challenges and obligations of living. They must learn the art of self-control. They should be equipped with the personal strength needed to meet the demands imposed on them by their school, peer groups, and later adult responsibilities."[12] Certainly these truths apply to healthy habits as well.

Dr. Dobson goes on to say that, "I believe that if it is desirable for children to be kind, appreciative, and pleasant, those qualities should be taught – not hoped for. If we want to see honesty, truthfulness, and unselfishness in our offspring, then these characteristics should be the conscious objectives of our early instructional process. If it is important to produce respectful, responsible, young citizens, then we should set out to mold them accordingly. The point is obvious: *heredity does not equip a child with proper attitudes; children learn what they are taught.* We cannot expect the coveted behavior to appear magically if we have not done our early homework."[13]

There is a parallel between the preceding paragraphs by Dr. Dobson and the need to teach healthy lifestyle habits to our children. We do not just hope for essential characteristics, such as honesty and kindness, to develop in our children and then settle for whatever the results may be. We guide and direct our youngsters towards them. In the same way, if we want children to eat healthfully, we must educate them about a nutritious diet. If we desire for them to enjoy and engage in physical activity, we have to show them how to do so. If we simply hope for these things, they will not materialize. Because it is important to produce healthy, fit, vibrant citizens, we must train kids how to become – and stay – this way.

While genetics may influence a child's tendency towards a certain body size and/or health status, heredity does not have the final say. If we teach healthy habits to our children, they will acquire them, just as they learn to share with others or not to throw food at the dinner table. And these beneficial habits will have a far greater impact on a child's health and weight than genetics alone. Healthy habits will not just suddenly appear in our kids. We have to teach them and be positive role models, just as we have to provide guidance and set good examples if we desire for our youngsters to develop admirable character traits, such as patience and selflessness.

In *What Every Mom Needs,* Elisa Morgan and Carol Kuykendall explain that moms need to start teaching very young children, even toddlers, to help around the house: "Sure, we can't expect our little ones to learn it all now, but now is the time to start. Cooking, cleaning, and washing clothes are skills that are best taught by instruction and repetition. A child doesn't automatically begin to exercise these skills when he or she turns eighteen. We help them out by beginning to teach them now (before they become moody teenagers!). Not only will it make their lives easier as adults, but it will also influence who they become as grown people, for their families and for the larger world they inhabit."[14] It is exactly the same with healthy habits.

At times, it will be helpful to explain to a child precisely why it is important to eat healthy, or the specific reasons that it is better to go outside and run around rather than watch another TV show. This is an ideal learning opportunity for a youngster. For instance, we can emphasize how fruits and vegetables make our bodies healthy and less likely to get sick, and that physical activity helps us feel good and keeps our bodies strong. Try never to miss a teachable moment – a simple explanation about the "why" really does motivate young ones to want to take care of themselves and their bodies.

Parents Must be Encouraged to Seek Help

As previously stated, adults – specifically parents – are responsible for preventing and reversing childhood obesity and chronic disease. A discouraging reality is that surprisingly few – about one out of every ten – parents referred for nutrition counseling for their child's weight actually schedule and attend an appointment. Unfortunately, this is not an exaggeration.

So the first issue is encouraging parents to seek help for an overweight child. Why do many appear to be unconcerned? It is usually because parents do not comprehend the gravity of the problem, or the absolute necessity of addressing it immediately. Complicating the matter is that oftentimes adults struggle with our own weight issues. Thus, change must begin with the parents and in the family. If family members neglect to change lifestyle habits in an effort to improve our own health, it will be impossible for a child to do so.

In fact, research has proven that children with overweight or obese parents are much more likely to become overweight or obese themselves.[15,16] One study found that the risk of obesity in adulthood more than doubled for children under ten who had at least one obese parent.[17] This is likely due to a combination of genetic and environmental factors, not merely one or the other. Consequently, these children are of particular concern, and we must be even more vigilant to prevent and treat weight issues in these kids, from the very beginning of their lives.

In regards to genetic predisposition and the prevention of obesity, consider an otherwise healthy individual with a strong family history of heart disease. As a result, she would be at a higher risk of developing heart disease. If she was determined to prevent it, she would modify her lifestyle – largely through diet and exercise. In the same way, those who have inherited a tendency to become overweight – individuals who have a family history, such as at least one overweight parent – must modify lifestyle behaviors and habits in order to prevent themselves from becoming overweight.

American youths need your help. Whatever your involvement with a child – a parent, guardian, relative, family friend, mentor, teacher, coach, caregiver, Sunday school teacher, youth leader, pediatrician, medical professional, public health employee, social worker, etcetera – the future of America needs your help, literally. Parents and guardians of children and adolescents who are overweight need to be encouraged to seek help for that child immediately. In most cases, and especially if at least one parent is overweight, that child will not outgrow his weight issue; his weight status, along with his health, will only continue to worsen. Adults cannot remain silent and act as though everything is going to be okay, because it may not. This requires collective, community-wide efforts. The obesity epidemic cannot be fought by medical and public health professionals alone, but if we all join together – with everyone's help – there is hope.

Weight is certainly a sensitive topic, but there are gentle and appropriate ways to approach it with a parent or guardian. Most importantly, make sure that the child is not present and cannot overhear the conversation. One option is to start by mentioning topics discussed in this book, especially the health consequences of obesity and the importance of seeking help for children right away. Explain that the subject is being broached solely out of care for the child and concern about her health (not her weight). If it is appropriate and not awkward, ask if the child is being followed by a healthcare professional, such as a doctor, registered dietitian, or nurse practitioner. If not, inquire about the parent's willingness to take her to a medical specialist with expertise in this area. Be careful to tread lightly, but do not be afraid of offending the parent – a child's life is at stake, after all. If all else fails or it is too uncomfortable, simply recommend this book as a reference for the parent or guardian.

Generational Cycle Must be Broken

Childhood and adult obesity can be compared to a generational cycle. Although we rarely admit it, detrimental family cycles do exist today. Examples include alcoholism, drug addiction, incarceration, abuse, poverty, teenage pregnancy, dropping out of school, and so on. Oftentimes these patterns become a family cycle – something that is passed on and repeated from generation to generation.

Obesity has become a similar issue. Until someone in the family steps up and says, "No, I am not going to succumb to this problem that has plagued my family for decades," it is going to continue to occur from generation to generation. No cycle is easy to break; ingrained, unhealthy habits are difficult to put an end to, but the good news is that it *is* possible. Unhealthy family cycles are defeated by brave individuals every day – many have family members or friends we deeply admire for doing so in their own families. Obesity is one of those cycles to which we have to step up and say, "No more." Americans must take a stance against unhealthy lifestyle habits, obesity, and chronic illness in our families.

Parents Must be Present to Train Children

A primary goal of parenting is to set our children up to win; we desire the very best for our kids. This goal should encompass every area of their lives, including their health and well-being. But because we are not adequately training our children, we are setting them up to fail in this area, and to fail miserably. The epidemic of obesity in our nation makes the truth painfully obvious: we have done an enormous disservice to our children.

In their book, *What Every Child Needs,* mothering experts Elisa Morgan and Carol Kuykendall admit that, "Maintaining the physical place called home is a challenge these days. Jobs, sports, even hobbies often take higher priority in some families." Notwithstanding, they continue: "Child advocate Marian Wright Edelman emphasizes the importance of a home. 'Parents for today's children must at all cost maintain a home, a center of love for their nurture and security. The pressure of our high-powered civilization is too much for a homeless and loveless child. . . *Nothing* must separate parents from their duty to their children."[18,19]

In order to train our children, parents must be present – we must be there for them and we must spend time with them. Synonyms for the word "train" in its verb tense include: teach, instruct, prepare, guide, coach, educate, and tutor.[20] This is an obligation that parents cannot pass on to others. For example, school systems and teachers have the task of helping train children academically; they are not accountable for educating children in other areas of life – that is a parent's job. Teachers may be able to reinforce what parents teach at home, but with overflowing classrooms of children in their care, it is impossible for them to take responsibility. In a child's life, there is no substitute for the time and attention of a mother and father.

Parents cannot train children to be healthy in every area of life – physically, emotionally, relationally, spiritually, and so forth – if we are not present. Parents should carefully review the preceding synonyms of the word "train," and bear in mind that we are called to do this in every area of our children's lives. Regardless of excuses, the bottom line is that if we are not present in our children's lives – if we are not teaching them healthy habits – then we are not fulfilling our role as parents, which is one of the greatest duties with which we have been charged.

Quantity and Quality Time

Spending time with our children is vital in order to demonstrate our love for them, as well as to train them. This refers to both the quantity and quality of the time – there is a considerable difference between the two. Sitting for hour upon hour in front of the television with our children may comprise quantity time, but it definitely does not represent quality time. One half-hour of playing catch or riding bikes with our children is much better than spending hours sitting in front of the television or running errands in the car with them. However, one half-hour of play time does not qualify as quantity time. Children need to spend ample amounts of time, including quality moments, with their parents in order to be effectively trained by them.

Parents Must be Good Role Models

Children are trained largely by example – by watching their parents and other adult family members, such as grandparents, aunts, and uncles. In fact, whether we realize it or not, we often parent more by example than with our words. Children internalize the things that adults do, the way we act, the things we say, the habits we have developed. Adults are role models for children in every area of life, including the development of healthy habits.

Positive or negative, parents and family members have a significant influence on how children and adolescents eat. For example, the food choices that parents make have been shown to affect the food preferences of our kids.[21] This is because impressionable youngsters glean preferences, attitudes, and values about food and eating habits from interactions with their family.[22] Moreover, the food preferences of a child's family members determine which foods and beverages are available in the home.

Because parents strongly affect children's and adolescent's food preferences, it is critical that we be highly aware of the ways we portray the foods we like and dislike. It is not uncommon to encounter a parent who, while sitting with their child in a nutrition counseling session, states, "Yuck, I do not like tomatoes," as an extremely unpleasant look crosses her face. This has occurred even when the child has already admitted, "Oh, I love tomatoes," or, "Yes, I am willing to try tomatoes." It is imperative that adults never complain about any type of food in front of a child; this is especially true in regards to a highly nutritious food, such as a fruit or vegetable.

Children are easily influenced. After hearing his mother or father complain about a food, it is nearly guaranteed that he will never try that particular food; further, he is certain to adopt a dislike for that food himself, even if he might actually enjoy it. For instance, my mom occasionally made rhubarb pie when I was a child. However, my dad absolutely detests rhubarb, and he made it abundantly clear to the entire family. Thankfully it is not a "super food" like broccoli or spinach, because even now, more than twenty years later, I cannot eat rhubarb. I distinctly remember sitting at the kitchen table and registering my dad's look of repulsion as his words of disgust rang in my ears. So I, of course, also refused to eat the pie. If my father disliked it so adamantly, I was convinced that there was no way I would sample it, much less enjoy it. To this day, I have never tried a bite of rhubarb, nor do I plan on ever doing so. This story is demonstrates the lasting impression that parents leave on our children.

More than that, when an adult openly expresses an aversion to a certain food, it gives youngsters permission to do the same. The thought process is: "My mom does not enjoy or consume broccoli, so it is acceptable for me to dislike and refuse to eat spinach." Parents already face numerous obstacles in convincing children to eat healthful, well-balanced meals; we need not provide them with further justification for being picky eaters.

While it may be tempting to convey to children, "Do as I say, not as I do," it is counterproductive. If youth observe adults skipping breakfast, avoiding vegetables, picking up fast-food, or snacking on candy, we cannot expect them to do anything but the same. If our favorite place is on the couch in front of the television instead of outside taking a walk or at the gym working out, kids certainly cannot be expected to go outside and play rather than watch TV or play video games.

While the list goes on and on, setting a good example for children and adolescents means eating well and not buying unwholesome foods in the first place; it refers to consuming a variety of fruits and vegetables and avoiding excessive amounts of fat, sugar, and sodium; it also includes not having "junk food" readily available in the house or frequenting the local fast-food drive through. Additionally, being a positive role model involves being physically active on a regular basis and including our children when appropriate, as well as limiting our "screen time" and getting plenty of sleep. The bottom line is that as a parent, relative, or mentor with an unhealthy habit of any kind, whether it be smoking, using bad language, watching too much television, not wearing a seatbelt, making unwise food choices, or being physically inactive, it is critical to make changes for the sake of the children that are watching us, if not ourselves, today.

Children Must be A Top Priority

Parents need to decide what – or, better yet, who – is more important: ourselves, our busy lives, and our hectic schedules or our children and their health, well-being, and quality of life. If we truly value our children's short- and long-term health, we will take the time and energy required to ensure that they lead a healthy life, as detailed in the following chapters. This includes breastfeeding our babies; preparing wholesome baby and toddler foods; instilling positive eating and physical activity habits early on; serving a healthy breakfast; preparing nourishing lunches; offering wholesome snacks; decreasing consumption of restaurant foods; cooking and sitting down to nutritious family dinners; being physically active as a family; insisting that children be more active; limiting the amount of time our families spend in front of technological devices and screens; and ensuring that every family member gets adequate sleep, rest, and relaxation.

When it comes down to it, humans make time for what we value. If, as a parent, we do not have time to pack a healthy lunch for our child on most days of the week, or to prepare and sit down to a well-balanced family dinner more evenings than not, we are probably too busy and/or need to closely examine our priorities. The same is true if we are unable to offer a wholesome breakfast or serve nourishing snacks. Other obligations have been put ahead of our duty as parents. Parents in our country must re-evaluate our priorities, and family should be at the top – not only in word, but in action as well. As parents, one of our first and most important responsibilities is our children. Prospective parents need to consider this, too: When planning to have children, be prepared to make them an utmost priority and do all that is required to help them lead a healthy life.

Children become a top priority when we put them at the number one spot on our "things to do" list. The opportunities for spending quality and quantity time with our kids on a daily basis are endless.

- Simply hang out and converse with them – spend more time listening than talking.

- Get out and be active together, such as by taking a walk or going to the park.

- Prepare and eat nutritious meals with our children.

- Plan and pack wholesome lunches with and for them.

- Teach youngsters how to cook healthfully.

- Play board games as a family.

- Sit down and help kids with their homework.

- Complete a craft or other project with each other.

- Volunteer at our children's schools and in their classrooms.

- Attend a community, sporting, or other event together.

- Additional suggestions will be found in the final sections of chapters nine and ten, "Establishing Physical Activity Habits Early" and "Too Much Screen Time."

Invest in a child and the dividends reaped by all – both now and in the future – will be incalculable. This book, and specifically this chapter, is not meant to discourage or criticize American parents – quite the opposite, in fact; it is intended to educate, inspire, and motivate – to arouse parents in this nation to take action.

Now that it has been established that the family, especially parents, carries the majority of responsibility for our children's health, we will examine specific ways that this can be followed through upon, starting with breastfeeding.

3 BREASTFEEDING IS THE BEST START

Jenna's mom is keenly aware of the countless benefits of breastfeeding, and she is happy to take advantage of each one. In her mind, however, there is one benefit that supersedes them all: the prevention of obesity. Even though Jenna is only a newborn and there is no way to know whether or not she might become overweight, Jenna has a strong family history of obesity so her mother wants to do all that she can to protect Jenna. Jenna's mother herself is obese, and Jenna's older brother, although only three years old, is already overweight. Jenna has an obese grandfather and two overweight grandmothers, as well as a number of overweight and obese aunts, uncles, and cousins. Therefore, Jenna's mom is intent on breastfeeding her for as long as possible.

It cannot be overlooked that as the problem of overweight and obesity worsens in our country, rates of breastfeeding are far less than ideal. This is despite the fact that public health authorities worldwide, including the American Academy of Pediatrics (AAP) and the World Health Organization (WHO), strongly endorse breastfeeding. In fact, "The American Academy of Pediatrics recognizes that breastfeeding is important for the optimal health and development of infants and children."[1] Furthermore, the AAP acknowledges that breastfeeding helps achieve the most favorable health, developmental, and psychosocial outcomes for a baby.[2]

As such, the AAP recommends breastfeeding as the sole source of nutrition for the first six months of life (no water, formula, other liquids, or solid foods), and thereafter, breast milk along with solid foods until at least twelve months of age; after twelve months, the continuation of breastfeeding is recommended for as long as both mother and child desire.[3] In order to take advantage of breast milk's nutritional and immunological properties, the WHO recommends exclusive breastfeeding (no water, formula, other liquids, or solid foods) for a baby's first six months, then continued breastfeeding in combination with solid foods until the child is at least two years old.[4]

Inadequate Rates of Breastfeeding

Historically, women who lived in traditional hunter and gatherer cultures breastfed each of their children for two to three years.[5] In colonial America, mothers usually breastfed their babies through at least two summers.[6] However, as society became more modernized and industrialized, breastfeeding waned in popularity. Today, much more is known about the benefits of breastfeeding and the unique properties of human milk, yet breastfeeding rates in America remain inadequate. On a positive note, though, the number of breastfed babies has been steadily growing over time, largely due to increased public health efforts promoting the benefits of mother's milk. While considerable work remains in order to bring breastfeeding rates up to adequate levels, it can be done. Much of this involves convincing parents-to-be that, indeed, babies are born to be breastfed.

Babies Were Born to Be Breastfed

In 2004, the United States Department of Health and Human Services and the Advertising Council launched the National Breastfeeding Awareness Campaign, a public health campaign designed to promote breastfeeding. The goal was to increase breastfeeding rates and support in the United States. The campaign included print, television, and radio advertisements. These public service announcements were creative, outside-the-box, and quite different from what had been done before. Rather than simply emphasizing the benefits of breastfeeding, the campaign alluded to the risks of not breastfeeding. The tag line of the announcements was "Babies were born to be breastfed." The ads also addressed the importance of breastfeeding exclusively for the first six months.

The print advertisements highlighted breastfeeding's role in reducing a child's risk of respiratory illness, ear infections, and obesity; the fourth ad simply stated: "Babies were born to be breastfed" (please refer to Figures 1 through 4). There were also two television commercials. One showed two pregnant women log-rolling, the other presented a pregnant woman riding a mechanical bull. Both ads asked: "You wouldn't take risks before your baby's born . . . Why start after?" Each TV commercial ended with the message: "Recent studies show babies who are breastfed are less likely to develop ear infections, respiratory illnesses, and diarrhea. Babies were born to be breastfed." Two radio announcements stressed the relationship between breastfeeding and protection against illness, specifically the decreased risk of ear infections and respiratory illness. The end of each radio spot specified that, "Babies were born to be breastfed exclusively for six months."

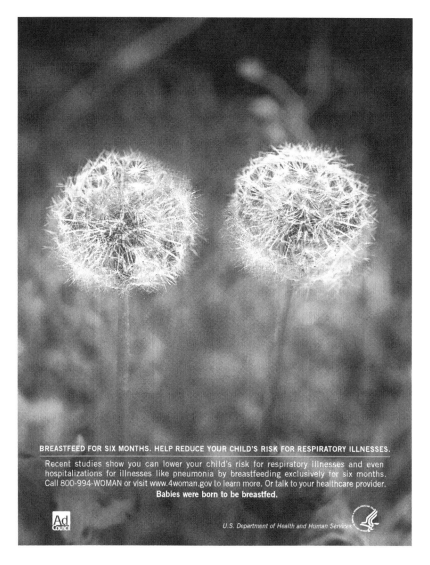

Figure 1: National Breastfeeding Awareness Campaign Print Advertisement: Respiratory Illness[6]

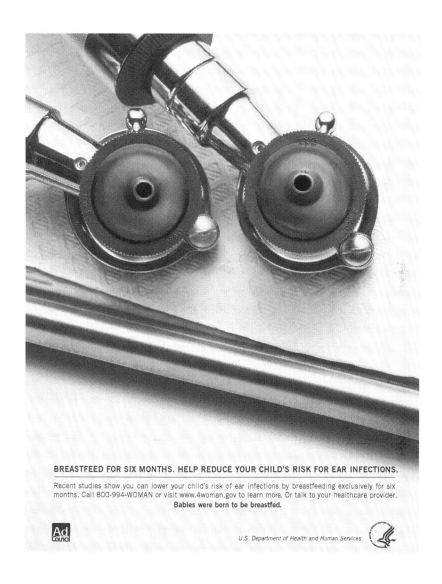

Figure 2: National Breastfeeding Awareness Campaign Print Advertisement: Ear Infections[7]

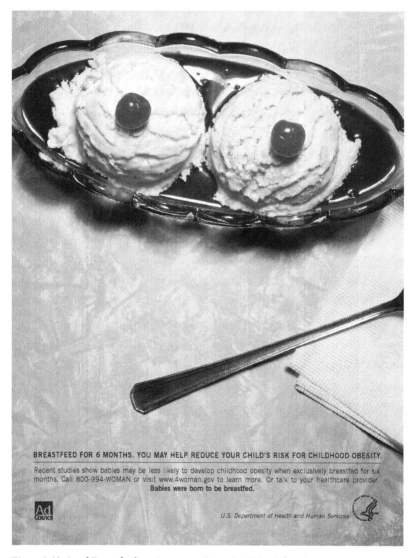

Figure 3: National Breastfeeding Awareness Campaign Print Advertisement: Childhood Obesity[8]

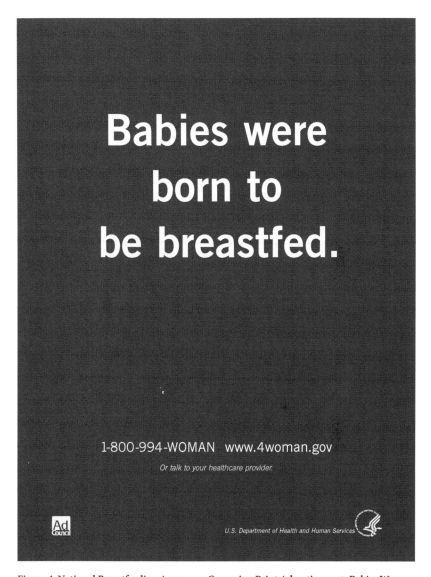

Figure 4: National Breastfeeding Awareness Campaign Print Advertisement: Babies Were Born to Be Breastfed[9]

As you read this chapter, please keep in mind that if you did not breastfeed and currently have an overweight child or adolescent, hope is not lost. There are plenty of other opportunities for improving your child's health and weight status. If, however, you are pregnant, thinking about becoming pregnant, or have a newborn, it would be wise to seriously consider breastfeeding. There are far too many benefits not to do so. Concerning the prevention of overweight and obesity, if at least one of your child's parents is overweight or has a family history of obesity, breastfeeding is undoubtedly the best option. If a family history of weight issues is not necessarily a concern, the numerous advantages of breastfeeding still make it inconceivable to bypass this once-in-a-lifetime opportunity. Besides, even though your child may not have a genetic predisposition for obesity, that does not guarantee that he or she is immune to the possibility, especially considering the path away from healthy lifestyle habits on which our nation is currently travelling.

The Benefits of Breastfeeding

The benefits of breastfeeding cannot be overstated, and this is true in respect to both the baby and the mother. There are countless benefits – some are immediate, some long-term, and some are both. It is highly probable that there are advantages of which we are not even aware because they have yet to be discovered, but research continues to provide convincing evidence that "breast is best." It is important to be aware that in the majority of studies regarding the positive effects of breastfeeding, breastfeeding exclusively and for a longer duration yielded the greatest benefits; that is, solely breastfeeding without giving any formula, water, juice, or other foods until the baby is at least six months of age appears to be the most advantageous.

Benefits of Breastfeeding for Baby

Ideal Source of Nutrition

First and foremost, breast milk is the ideal source of nutrition for a baby.[11] God designed it that way. It provides the perfect amount of fat, protein, carbohydrates, fluid, vitamins, and minerals needed for the optimal growth and development of an infant. In fact, the *New Mother's Guide to Breastfeeding* by the American Academy of Pediatrics says, "Breast milk is such a rich, nourishing mixture that scientists have yet to identify all of its elements; no formula manufacturer has managed or will ever be able to fully replicate it."[12] More than that, the composition of breast milk actually changes over time in order to provide the nutrients that a growing baby requires at each stage of development.[13] Likewise, the components in a mother's milk adjust throughout the day in order to meet her baby's needs, and the amount of fat in breast milk increases during a feeding so that the infant feels full and satisfied at the end.[14,15] No formula is able to do that!

Well-Tolerated, Easy to Digest, and Safe

In addition to being the best form of nutrition, breast milk is well-tolerated and easy for a baby to digest – much more so than any formula available.[16] Formula-fed babies often experience painful digestive problems such as constipation, diarrhea, and/or reflux. This necessitates switching from formula to formula in order to find one that works, which is costly, time-consuming, and frustrating.

It can be difficult – if not impossible – to find a formula that a baby tolerates well, and he may end up requiring a specialized type, which is extremely expensive. With breastfeeding, none of this is necessary. Moreover, breast milk is safe. There is no need to question exactly what you are feeding your baby, nor fear that it might be recalled, as is the case with infant formulas.

Obesity Prevention

Most relevant to this book is the fact that research proves that breastfeeding prevents obesity.[17,18] Several studies demonstrate that breastfeeding results in lower rates of obesity in childhood, adolescence, and later in life.[19,20,21] Further, the longer a mother breastfeeds her infant, the more protection the baby receives against overweight and obesity.[22,23]

There are two main theories as to why breastfed babies are less likely to become overweight or obese. The first has to do with the remarkable composition and biological properties of breast milk. For instance, formula-fed babies consume more protein than breastfed babies, and it is believed that a high protein intake early in life may play a role in the development of obesity.[24] Another factor is that lower levels of insulin are found in babies who are breastfed compared to those who are formula-fed; this is significant because insulin is a hormone that stimulates the storage of fat.[25]

The second theory is related to the concept of infant versus parental feeding control. Breastfed infants stop nursing when they feel full and thus control their own intake. On the other hand, a bottle-fed infant's feeding tends to be more controlled by the parent or caregiver, which can lead to overfeeding.[26] For example, a mother encourages her baby finish off an entire eight-ounce bottle even though the child was truly full after drinking only six ounces. Because of this, bottle-fed babies may become desensitized to their internal hunger and fullness cues. Additionally, when breastfed babies begin to eat solids, there is a natural, steady decline in the amount of breast milk they consume.[27] Bottle-fed infants, however, are often given the same amount of formula, even after they have been introduced to solids. This, in turn, can result in overfeeding.

Immune Protection

As though the prevention of obesity alone is not sufficient, breastfeeding offers many additional health benefits to a baby. One major advantage is that breast milk contains antibodies, live white blood cells, enzymes, and other special immune factors which are passed from a mother to her baby.[28,29] This is beneficial for a newborn's immune system because he has never been exposed to germs, and these substances present in breast milk help him fight bacteria and viruses. Amazingly, breastfed babies experience fewer bouts of colds, vomiting, diarrhea, pneumonia, and ear infections as well as other illnesses and infections.[30,31] Another immunologic benefit of breastfeeding is that it reduces the likelihood of food and other allergies.[32,33,34]

Disease Prevention

More than that, breastfeeding prevents chronic disease: Babies who are breastfed have a decreased risk of many life-threatening illnesses as both a child and an adult.[35] Some of the diseases that breast milk guards against are type 1 and type 2 diabetes;[36,37,38] cardiovascular disease;[39,40] certain cancers, including childhood leukemia[41,42] and breast cancer in adult females;[43,44] asthma;[45,46] as well as some digestive disorders, such as Crohn's disease.[47,48] Incredibly, breastfeeding has even been found to lessen the incidence Sudden Infant Death Syndrome (SIDS)[49,50,51] and autism,[52,53] which is remarkable because much remains unknown about these conditions, including how to prevent them.

Brain Development

Breast milk promotes – even enhances – brain development.[54,55] Research reveals that children who were breastfed as babies score higher on IQ and other cognitive tests, regardless of factors such as socioeconomic status or mother's intelligence.[56,57,58] This is impressive. Not surprisingly, these children tend to be more successful in school.[59,60] As with most benefits of breastfeeding, the longer a mother breastfeeds her baby, the more significant the effects; additionally, these favorable outcomes are long-lasting, persisting into adolescence and even adulthood.[61,62] According to one study, compared to children breastfed for longer than six months, children breastfed fewer than three months were more likely to receive lower-than-average scores on cognitive tests at both one year and five years of age.[63]

Emotional Health

Endorphins, chemicals that help relieve stress, are present in breast milk at high amounts for the first few days after birth.[64] This may help newborns adjust to life outside of the womb. Research also indicates that children who were breastfed are better able to handle stress than those who were formula-fed, even after accounting for other factors that might be involved.[65] This does not necessarily mean that breast milk itself helps kids cope with anxiety. Researchers suggest that the physical and emotional closeness experienced by a mother and her baby while breastfeeding may play a role in the development of that child's stress-response. And that because breastfeeding strengthens the mother-child bond, it may in turn have long-term effects on the child's ability to deal with anxiety. Although the exact mechanisms might not be fully understood, it is apparent that children who were breastfed are less likely to be negatively impacted by stress and anxiety than those who were formula-fed.

Benefits of Breastfeeding for Mother

Weight Loss

There are numerous advantages of breastfeeding for a mother as well. One that is vitally important to a woman who has just given birth is returning to her pre-pregnancy weight. Breastfeeding facilitates weight loss in at least three ways: it speeds the return of the uterus to its normal size (which also helps decrease bleeding after a baby is born), it enhances a woman's metabolism, and it burns calories.[66,67] Breastfeeding actually requires more calories than pregnancy.

Mother-Baby Bond

Another critical concern for a new mom is the bond she forms with her baby, and breastfeeding serves to enhance this bond.[68] Breastfeeding fosters physical contact and emotional attachment which are very important for a newborn and help her feel more secure, warm, and comforted.[69,70] Mothers experience fulfillment and joy from the physical and emotional closeness that breastfeeding allows.[71,72] And as a baby becomes older and more independent, such as being able to crawl around on her own, the intimacy of breastfeeding becomes even more meaningful for a mom.

Disease Prevention

Breastfeeding also aids in disease prevention – not just for the baby, but for a mother as well. For example, research demonstrates that moms who breastfeed their babies decrease their chances of developing breast and ovarian cancer.[73,74] In fact, researchers estimate that there would be 250 thousand fewer cases of breast cancer diagnosed per year in the United States if every mother breastfed each of her babies for six months longer than she originally intended.[75] This is significant considering that breast cancer is on the rise among women of all ages and we have become desperate to prevent it. Breastfeeding may also reduce the risk of other cancers, including uterine, endometrial, and thyroid, but more research is needed in this area.

Women who breastfeed also lower their risk of cardiovascular disease, high blood pressure, and even type 2 diabetes.[76,77,78] Moreover, the longer a woman breastfeeds, the more protection she gains.[79,80] This is important because cardiovascular disease, for which high blood pressure and diabetes are risk factors, is a leading health concern and major cause of death among women – but it is also highly preventable.[81]

Further, it appears that breastfeeding contributes to a higher bone mineral density, which protects against the development of osteoporosis and bone fractures later in life.[82,83] Similar to breast cancer and cardiovascular disease, this is worth noting because low bone mineral density and osteoporosis occur all too commonly in older women, and women of all ages are striving to improve their bone health in an effort to prevent osteoporosis.

Emotional Health

Beyond physical health, breastfeeding seems to improve a woman's emotional well-being. Studies reveal that breastfeeding moms tend to experience more positive moods as well as less stress, anxiety, and depression than mothers that formula-feed.[84,85] It has also been found that women who breastfeed feel closer to their babies than those who do not.[86] The association between breastfeeding and emotional health may, at least in part, be related to the hormones prolactin and oxytocin, which circulate at high levels in a breastfeeding woman.[87,88]

Saves Time, Energy, and Money

Practically-speaking, breastfeeding saves time and money. It is much more cost-effective and convenient than formula, which is expensive and takes time and effort to prepare. Unlike bottle-feeding, you do not have to purchase bottles, nipples, bottle warmers, or bottle brushes when you breastfeed. Breast milk is always ready and available; it saves time and energy because there is no need to sterilize bottles or water, not to mention mix or warm the formula.

Moreover, when a child is breastfed, he typically does not need to be weaned from a bottle, which simplifies and makes life more pleasant for everyone. Many exclusively breastfed infants rarely require a bottle, so they do not become attached to it like those who are formula-fed. When it is time, breastfed babies typically take fluids from a cup rather than a bottle without complaining.

The fact that a breastfed baby does not usually grow attached to a bottle decreases the likelihood that she will be overweight as a toddler. Many overweight toddlers become that way – largely, if not entirely – because of an excessive intake of milk and/or juice from the bottle. It is true that children need to consume an adequate amount of dairy products each day, and those under two should be drinking whole milk. However, it is not necessary or healthful for toddlers to consume bottles full of high-calorie liquids all throughout the day. In fact, when young children do so, their little stomachs become so full of fluids that they have no appetite for the healthy, nutrient-rich foods they need.

Conversely, when children take liquids from a cup, they naturally drink less than if they were to take them from a bottle. Even a toddler who was accustomed to a bottle from birth consumes a smaller amount of liquid once he is weaned to a cup, partly because he is eating more solid foods. In addition, toddler cups usually hold fewer fluid ounces than bottles, and parents do not normally fill them to the top as they tend to do with bottles. What is more, cups are not as easy or comforting for children to use as bottles.

Why Not Breastfeed?

In many cases, breastfeeding is not entirely simple or stress-free during the initial days after birth, especially with the first baby. It can definitely be a challenge early on. If breastfeeding issues do arise, however, lactation consultants are available at most hospitals and public health clinics to help new mothers work through any problems rather than simply quit – or decide not to attempt – breastfeeding altogether. It is essential for a new mom to have a knowledgeable and experienced individual to provide support and encouragement, as well as practical assistance and advice, particularly at a time when she may begin to doubt her ability to breastfeed. Breastfeeding does become easier over time – much easier. After the first challenging days, weeks, possibly even months, it becomes like second nature for both mother and child. This is not to insinuate that breastfeeding is always effortless, because it does require time and energy. Quite simply, though, breastfeeding is God's design.

Without a doubt, breastfeeding confers numerous benefits to a baby and mother. However, stated another way, there are risks inherent to not breastfeeding. Rather than simply affirming that there are positive outcomes related to breastfeeding, it can also be said that there may be adverse consequences of not breastfeeding. For example, as discussed earlier, babies who are not breastfed are at an increased risk of immediate health concerns, including gastrointestinal problems, colds, ear infections, and allergies. Further, over the long-term, children who were not breastfed during infancy have a greater chance of medical issues, such as obesity, diabetes, heart disease, cancer, and asthma. Thus, because of the consequences associated with not breastfeeding, any substitute for mother's milk could be considered potentially noxious to a baby's health and well-being, whether or not it directly causes problems for an infant. Conversely, breast milk could be viewed as a life-giving antidote.

Amidst the multitude of advantages already known about breastfeeding, researchers continue to discover additional benefits. Considering the countless positive outcomes – for both baby and mama – only one question remains: Why not breastfeed? Regardless of the plethora of infant formulas currently on the market and the claims that are made for them, the AAP states: "It is impossible to perfectly mimic a substance as complex as human breast milk."[89] Therefore, America needs to become a society where breastfeeding is the standard, the norm, the expectation. After all, "Babies were born to be breastfed." The next step in preventing obesity and promoting health is establishing healthy eating habits – and doing so early in life. This is explained in detail in the following chapter.

4 HEALTHY EATING HABITS BEGIN EARLY

Joey is a two-and-a-half year old with doggedly strong food preferences. He refuses to eat many foods, especially fresh fruits and vegetables. Ever since he began eating solid foods at about six months of age, he has been on a steady diet of highly processed foods, usually directly out of some sort of package. One of his first foods was infant cereal mixed with fruit, which was sweet to his taste buds. Soon after, he was introduced to jarred fruit mixtures, which are also naturally sweet. For vegetables, Joey was typically served sweet varieties or combinations containing fruit, so again, he grew increasingly accustomed to sweet flavors. He refused to eat green beans the first time his mom offered them, so she never tried to feed him a green vegetable again. Joey was also introduced to dessert items early on. Now at two-and-a-half, Joey prefers pre-packaged toddler meals rather than fresh, natural foods. Snack time is more of the same: he is typically given a packaged item containing little nutritional value, like crackers or cookies, puffs, chewy fruit treats, or a cereal bar. Joey's mother cannot remember the last time he ate a non-starchy green vegetable or piece of fresh fruit other than a banana. But it is not that she is an irresponsible mother, or that she is not striving to do the very best for her young son. Joey's mom has been diligent about bathing him daily and teaching him to brush his teeth at least twice a day; she has conscientiously taught him to be respectful and has trained him to always say "please" and "thank you." The fact of the matter is that no one taught her to eat healthfully beginning at an early age, and now she is unaware of the necessity to do so for her child.

Research reveals that the path to obesity often begins as early as infancy and toddlerhood; already by the young age of two, children are forming habits that can make them more – or less – likely to be overweight or obese.[1,2] Lifestyle habits developed during childhood often become lifelong habits. More to the point, a child begins to establish eating patterns early in life, and these habits tend to persist long-term.[3,4] It has been suggested that some eating habits start to take shape before a child is even two years old.[5] Further, food preferences established during childhood not only influence future food choices, but can impact both immediate and long-term health, including the development of obesity.[6]

What is more, research shows that overweight toddlers and preschoolers do not necessarily outgrow their "baby fat" and are at a high risk of being overweight as older children. According to a National Institute of Child Health and Human Development study, children who are overweight at the age of two, three, or four-and-a-half are more than five times more likely to be overweight at twelve years of age than those who do not experience overweight in their younger years.[7] Toddlers and preschoolers who are at-risk of overweight are also more likely to be overweight at twelve years old.

Thus, it is critical that the development of healthy eating habits start when children are very young – even as soon as infancy.[8,9] Interestingly, research has found that parents and the family environment influence a child's eating habits as early as infancy.[10] And as Dr. Ruth Peters says in her book, *It's Never Too Soon to Discipline*, "As in many areas of life, a habit begun early is easier to establish and tends to remain longer than one started later."[11] That is why it is imperative to introduce healthy habits to children when they are young. Do we ignore the necessity of teaching our youngest ones to brush their teeth daily? What about the routine of bathing? It should be the same with eating habits, another foundational life skill. It is never too early to begin teaching children to eat a wholesome, nutritious diet. Peggy Frezon's story at the beginning of chapter two demonstrates the critical need for parents to fulfill this obligation. If Peggy's son, Andy, had been taught to eat healthfully early on, he probably would not have experienced a health scare at eighteen years of age. Children are more likely to adopt and practice beneficial eating habits throughout their lifetime if parents feed them a nutritious diet and teach them to eat wholesome foods beginning in infancy and toddlerhood, and continuing on through childhood and adolescence.

Paying Attention to Hunger and Fullness Cues

Perhaps one of the most effective ways to help children develop proper eating habits is by allowing and encouraging them to pay attention to their internal hunger and fullness cues. This is especially critical during infancy and early childhood. If children establish this practice in their younger years, they are likely to remain sensitive to their hunger and fullness signals as they get older, making it less likely that they will develop a tendency to overeat.

Children, particularly babies and toddlers, are quite in tune with their physiological hunger and fullness cues. They will eat only if and when they are hungry, not because the clock indicates that it is lunchtime. And once they are full, youngsters refuse to take another bite.

However, as children grow older, they often lose this sensitivity for a variety of reasons. First of all, society has trained us to ignore our hunger cues. We eat according to the clock; breakfast, lunch, and dinner are usually eaten at specific times rather than when the stomach growls. Additionally, families tend to be busy with a schedule that lacks flexibility, so children are forced to eat when there is time rather than when they are physiologically hungry. And once they start school, kids do not have a choice. They must eat breakfast in time to get out the door in the morning, and snack and lunch are eaten at prescribed times during the school day, whether or not they are hungry.

Further, families rarely sit down for regular family dinners anymore, which is addressed in chapter seven, "More Family Meals, Less Happy Meals®." It is impossible to sense the body's feelings of hunger and fullness when we are on-the-go. We tend to consume whatever is in front of us when we eat on-the-run, even if we are not truly hungry for every bite. And when we just graze haphazardly throughout the day, rather than slowing and sitting down for meals, our body may never actually feel hungry or satisfied. This often results in the consumption of a greater amount of food – and usually less wholesome food – over the course of a day than if we actually sat down to eat meals.

Unknowingly, parents and caregivers have negatively influenced children by insisting that: "You cannot leave the table until you finish your meal," or, "You must eat all of that if you want dessert." By demanding that children eat every last morsel of food on their plate, even if they are already full, we train children to ignore their inborn signals of satiety. Eventually this becomes a habit, resulting in a tendency to overeat. Over time, a child loses the ability to distinguish if he is satisfied as opposed to stuffed.

Television and other distractions, such as video games and computers, have become commonplace during mealtimes. This is discussed in detail in chapter ten, "Too Much Screen Time"; however, the bottom line is that when these distractions occupy our minds during meals, feelings of hunger and fullness get ignored, which can result in overeating.

Our job as parents and caregivers is to encourage children to be responsive to their biological feelings of hunger and fullness and not to squelch them. Although it is tempting, avoid coaxing your baby to finish the last couple pieces of food left in the bowl if she is turning her head or otherwise refusing a bite as a means of saying, "I am full," or "All done." And as your child gets older, remind her to tune in to her internal hunger and fullness cues. Do not try to persuade her to eat if she is not hungry, or to finish all the food on her plate if she feels full. Ensure that your child eats regular well-balanced meals and snacks throughout the day (rather than eating haphazardly) because this will enable her to sense her feelings of hunger and fullness. Also, insist that she routinely sit down to family dinners and that all media distractions, such as the television, are turned off during mealtimes. These specific topics are discussed in subsequent chapters.

Beyond that, heeding a child's internal hunger and fullness cues means that parents and caregivers cannot feed infants and young children as a means of keeping them entertained, nor can we allow older children to eat out of boredom. While it is convenient, offering young ones bite after bite in order to keep them silent and content so we can shop, talk on the phone, or take care of other business teaches them to ignore their innate feeding signals. And the same is true if we allow children to eat when it is not meal or snack time and they are not actually hungry, but they are simply bored. In both of these cases, it may require creativity and imagination, but there are ways other than food to distract children and keep them occupied.

Limiting Sugar and Salt

The regular consumption of high-sugar, high-salt, and/or high-fat foods can lead to immediate health and weight issues among babies and young children. What is of more concern is that the eating habits established during these early stages may have serious long-term effects, whether or not there are immediate consequences. Many food preferences are formed early in life.[12,13] Hence, we broach a central point of this chapter: if we serve sugary, salty, and otherwise unhealthy foods to babies, toddlers, and young children, they will develop a preference for these foods and insist on a steady supply of highly-flavorful treats as they grow older. And not just for dessert, but for breakfast, lunch, dinner, and snack-time as well. This, in turn, sets them up for the possibility of developing of obesity and chronic diseases, such as type 2 diabetes and heart disease.

It is critical that infants and young children consume a wholesome, healthy diet every day – it may be more important at this stage in life than at any other. Babies under one year of age should never be served foods containing sugar or salt. Exposure to these ingredients should be extremely limited for toddlers up to two years old, and closely monitored even among three to five-plus year olds. There is no reason for young children to eat as poorly as adults. For example, what reason is there for offering French fries or chips to an infant? If he is not exposed to these unhealthy foods, he will be unaware of them and gladly accept a much more healthful plain, mashed-up baked potato. Not only are sugar and salt unhealthy for kids' little bodies, but they quickly acquire a taste for sugary and salty foods – preferences that will stay with them for a lifetime. Establishing healthy habits starts the day a child is born.

Children are born with an innate preference for sweet and salty flavors.[14] But if parents limit children's exposure to ingredients such as sugar and salt in their early years, youngsters are less apt to grow up virtually addicted to these tastes; moreover, they will enjoy and have an appreciation for the natural taste of foods. One way to ensure that children do not become accustomed to eating "junk food" is to limit their intake of items such as sweetened beverages, cookies, chips, French fries, and so on. In fact, in the early years, these types of items should be avoided altogether.

The Truth about Juice

Consider juice, for example. If little ones are allowed to carry around bottles or cups of juice (even one hundred percent juice without added sweeteners tastes very sweet), they are going to expect to snack on sugar-laden beverages or candy as they grow older. In truth, it is not necessary for babies, toddlers, or children to drink juice. One hundred percent fruit juice does contain vitamin C. But if a child eats a well-rounded diet, including a variety of foods and plenty of fruits and vegetables, she is consuming an adequate amount of vitamin C. In fact, as will be discussed further in chapter eight, "The Truth about Sweetened Beverages," the American Academy of Pediatrics states that compared to whole fruit, juice offers no nutritional advantage.[15] Babies get their vitamin C from breast milk (or formula). And if a young child really needs to obtain vitamin C from juice, she only requires a small amount of one hundred percent juice to fulfill her daily vitamin C requirement: two to four ounces, or one-fourth to one-half of a cup. No child needs to be drinking cups or bottles full of juice. Juice is high in sugar, which is not good for a child's body or teeth, plus it causes her to become accustomed to the flavor of sugar in general, and the taste of sweetened beverages in particular. We cannot expect a toddler or young child to prefer plain water when she is older if she is regularly served juice. Instead, children need to be offered plain water to drink.

There is nothing unique or novel about the juices that baby food companies manufacture. These juices contain virtually the same amount of sugar and vitamin C as regular one hundred percent fruit juice. Furthermore, the water and fruit juice blends made specifically for toddlers and preschoolers are simply another way for young ones to develop a taste for sugar, as well as distaste for plain water, at an early age. And this is a preference that they will not outgrow. Just like juice, these drinks contain unnecessary sugar and set children on a path to become addicted to sweetened beverages.

The simplest solution is to refrain from keeping juice (and other sweetened beverages) in the house. Do not introduce juice to babies or toddlers, but once a child is older and desires it, reserve juice for special occasions as a "treat." If babies and toddlers are not offered juice, they will not be aware that there is a better-tasting option available and will drink water instead; moreover, they will develop an appreciation for water and will not mind the taste of it as they get older. As children grow, however, they are bound to be served juice at their friend's house, at birthday parties, and so on. In order to help them understand why they are typically served water instead of juice at home, explain that too much juice is not good for their bodies and that water is the best option. And if juice and other sweetened beverages are not in the house for older children to drink, they will drink what is available: water. Not only is it more healthy, but water is less expensive, readily available, and requires no preparation.

Please refer to chapter eight, "The Truth about Sweetened Beverages," for a further discussion on juice and other beverages, including recommendations issued by the American Academy of Pediatrics.

The Feeding Infants and Toddlers Study

The Feeding Infants and Toddlers Study (FITS) reveals many compelling facts about how American youngsters between four and twenty-four months of age eat. For example, researchers discovered that children under the age of two are not consuming enough fruits and vegetables. Infants (over six months old) and toddlers should have at least five servings of fruits and vegetables each day, yet the number that are not ingesting any at all is alarming: approximately one-fourth to one-third of those between the ages of seven months and one-and-a-half years do not eat any vegetables in a day, and about the same proportion of seven month to two year olds do not eat any fruit.[16] A disconcerting finding is that French fries are the most common "vegetable" consumed by toddlers, and that over a quarter of nineteen to twenty-four month olds eat French fries or other fried potatoes on any given day.[17] The concern is that French fries should never be counted as a vegetable in the first place. The adulteration that a potato encounters in order to be served as a French fry entirely negates any potential benefits that consuming a potato may have offered.

In addition, the research demonstrates that young children have an excessive intake of sugar. It was found that nearly half of babies seven to eight months old eat some kind of dessert, sugar-laden treat, or sweetened beverage (fruit-flavored drinks and/or carbonated sodas).[18] And it gets worse as a baby gets older: by the time they are two years old, over sixty percent of toddlers consume baked desserts, twenty percent eat candy, and nearly half drink sweet fruit beverages and/or carbonated sodas. Taken together, almost all (more than ninety percent of) toddlers between nineteen and twenty-four months ingest at least one type of high-sugar treat.

Sodium intake is also high, particularly among toddlers, with more than a fourth of nineteen to twenty-four month olds eating salty snacks.[19,20] In addition to high-salt snacks, the consumption of processed meats (lunch meats, hot dogs, bacon, sausage, ham) appears to be high in young children, contributing excess sodium to their diets.[21,22]

According to FITS, a large proportion of the items fed to young children are unhealthy options, and many even qualify as "junk food."[23] For example, sweet beverages (fruit-flavored drinks, carbonated sodas), sweetened cereals, butter/margarine/oil, cookies, processed meats (lunch meats, hot dogs, sausage, bacon), and baked goods (cakes, pies) accounted for almost twenty percent of the total calories ingested by toddlers in this study.[24,25] Most of these items are highly processed and contain large amounts of sugar, salt, and/or unhealthy fats, but are low in valuable nutrients such as vitamins, minerals, and fiber.

Furthermore, researchers discovered that toddlers often consume inappropriate items at snack time.[26] For instance, cookies, chips, fruit drinks, and/or candy were commonly served as an afternoon snack to fifteen to twenty-four month old toddlers.[27,28] Infants and toddlers have small stomachs yet high calorie and nutrient needs; this necessitates that they eat small amounts frequently. Thus, parents and caregivers need to make the most of snack times and offer nutritious, wholesome choices.

The bottom line is that foods that are high in calories, sugar, salt, and/or unhealthy fats but low in essential nutrients, such as fiber, protein, vitamins, and minerals, are unacceptable for infants and toddlers, whose nutrient needs are especially high.[29] Researchers concluded that due to the rising rates of childhood obesity in this country, the current dietary patterns of infants and toddlers warrant substantial concern and attention.[30]

Recommendations from the Feeding Infants and Toddlers Study

The findings of the Feeding Infants and Toddlers Study led to new insights concerning how America's youngest are fed. The following recommendations are related to increasing fruit and vegetable intake, decreasing sugar and salt consumption, appropriate beverage choices, healthy snacks options, and family responsibility regarding the diets of infants and toddlers.

Fruits and Vegetables

- When a baby begins to eat solid foods, progressively offer a variety of fruits and vegetables each day. Focus on dark green, leafy and deep yellow vegetables as well as colorful fruits.[31]

- Regularly serve age- and developmentally-appropriate fruits and vegetables at snack time.[32]

Sugar and Salt

- Avoid or strictly limit serving desserts, sweets (such as candy), and sweetened beverages to infants and toddlers.[33]

- Do not add salt to foods prepared at home; avoid or limit items that are high in salt, including processed meats and salty snacks; offer more fresh fruits and vegetables.[34]

Beverages

- To prevent an excessive sugar and calorie intake, limit one hundred percent fruit juice and fruit-flavored drinks, which tend to replace more nutritious foods in the diet.[35]

- Water is a good choice for satisfying thirst, and it does not cause unnecessary sugar or calorie consumption.[36]

Snacks

- Delay introducing – as well as strictly limit exposure to – items high in calories, sugar, salt, and/or unhealthy fats yet low in vital nutrients; this is critical so that infants and toddlers do not develop a preference for these foods rather than healthier options.[37]

- Infants and toddlers should be served wholesome, nutritious snacks, such as age- and developmentally-appropriate fruits and vegetables, whole grains, and dairy products instead of high-calorie, high-sugar, high-salt and/or high-fat items like cookies, candy, chips, and French fries.[38]

Family Involvement

- The family's food choices strongly influence what is served to young children; therefore, it might be necessary to involve the whole family in forming healthy eating habits.[39]

- Parents and caregivers must take responsibility and offer nutritious, appropriate foods to infants and toddlers. Furthermore, the entire family may need to modify its eating habits since these impressionable little ones usually desire to eat the same foods as the rest of their family.[40]

Early Exposure to Healthy Foods

In order to instill healthy eating habits in children, it is critical to expose infants (older than six months of age), toddlers, and preschoolers to the taste and texture of a variety of nutritious foods, including fruits, vegetables, and whole grains. When youngsters are served wholesome, nutritious foods, they are more likely to eat these types of foods as they get older. Research shows that a child's food choices at the age of eight are related to his food preferences when he was a toddler or preschooler.[41] Furthermore, babies and toddlers who are served a variety of fruits and vegetables are likely to eat a wider array of these health-promoting foods as they grow older and begin to make some of their own food choices.

A child's willingness to try and accept new food flavors is strongly influenced by her feeding experiences early in life.[42] Oftentimes, babies (over six months) and young children need to be exposed to a new food multiple times before they will accept it – sometimes as many as eight to ten times; the more a child is exposed to a certain food, the more likely she is to try and accept it.[43,44] This has even been observed in five to seven year olds: after being exposed to raw red bell pepper for eight days, children increasingly ate and enjoyed the vegetable.[45] Therefore, it can be concluded that consistently exposing young children to a wide variety of foods and flavors increases the likelihood that they will sample and learn to like unfamiliar or novel foods. Another factor that affects a youngster's willingness to accept an item is socialization: A child is more apt to try a food if she observes an adult, such as a parent, eating it.[46]

So even if your child frowns and adamantly refuses when served broccoli, for instance, do not give up. Rather, try, try, try again! Offer it prepared in a different manner, such as raw instead of cooked (if age-appropriate), or vice versa. If he continues to reject it after multiple (at least ten) attempts, discontinue broccoli for a period of time. Re-introduce it again in the future, in a few weeks or so. However, there are some foods that a child will always refuse; we are all entitled to our likes and dislikes. But when he is older, the chance that your child will try a new, healthy food – and like it – is much higher if he is exposed to a variety of nutritious foods in a positive manner as a baby and young child. And even if your child dislikes broccoli throughout his entire childhood, he may eat and enjoy it as an adult if he is repeatedly exposed to it in an encouraging way during his younger years.

An illustration of the impact that repeated exposure can make is when my husband and I first introduced a vegetable – pureed green beans – to our six month old daughter. Up until then, she had only had breast milk and infant rice cereal – both sweet-tasting and delicious to her developing palate. As a result, she was not pleased with green beans. In fact, her reaction caused me to worry that something was wrong. The look of sheer horror on her face was beyond any expression I had ever seen her display. She protested violently, with cries and wails that were completely out of character for her. It was an unpleasant experience, to say the least. I was assured that there was no major concern – that she merely detested green beans – when she abruptly ended her objections the moment we interrupted her meal. Was it the bitter taste – the complete opposite of anything she had ever tasted? The new texture? It was probably a combination of both.

Much to my dismay, I knew we needed to continue our attempts at feeding her green beans for at least a few more days. If I had not observed it myself, I would not believe the progress that was made. The next day, she objected to the green beans, but not nearly as adamantly as on day one. By the third or fourth day, she ate them with almost no complaint at all. And after that, she accepted them as if they were her favorite food. She continues to eat green beans to this day. Had we given up on that first day we introduced green beans, she may never have eaten them again.

Soon after, a sweet family came to me for nutrition counseling with their thirteen month old son who had a diagnosis of failure-to-thrive. He was underweight and malnourished, partly due to multiple food allergies. However, as I questioned these parents about their toddler's diet, I learned that his primary source of nutrition was sweet potatoes from a baby food jar; his parents explained that this was practically the only item he would eat. As I tried to determine why this young child would only eat jarred sweet potatoes, I ruled out all other possible factors – food allergies, texture issues, swallowing problems. In the end, it came down to one simple reason: when these parents began to introduce new foods to their son, he would not accept anything the first time it was offered. If he refused to eat something when they initially served it to him, they never gave it to him again. Over time, they began giving him the one and only item he would readily eat: sweet potatoes out of a baby food jar. So at thirteen months of age, that was the only food this child liked.

Because of an innocent mistake, these parents and their little boy had suffered. This family had to start back at square one with their one year old, which was not easy to do. Much frustration could have been avoided if this child had been offered foods – even the ones he did not accept the first few times – over and over again when he first began eating solids. Besides that, his diet would have been much more extensive and his issues of being underweight and malnourished would not have been as severe. In fact, as soon as this child's diet started to expand, he began to gain weight and become healthier.

These stories illustrate how easy it can be to neglect exposing our youngest, most impressionable ones to a variety of foods, particularly fruits and vegetables. Yet at the same time, it is absolutely critical to do so – and to do it over and over again.

Homemade Baby Food

Although it undoubtedly takes a little more time and effort, there are numerous advantages to preparing homemade food for your baby. Take, for example, one study that analyzed the sugar and sodium content of commercially prepared baby and toddler foods. Of the one hundred and eighty-six foods studied, sixty-three percent (one hundred and eighteen) had a high sugar and/or sodium content.[47] Researchers found that more than half of the products were high in sugar, which included items manufactured for toddlers as well as those produced specifically for infants. Products that tend to be especially high in sugar include desserts, teething biscuits, cookies, fruit snacks, yogurt snacks, and cereals (including cereal bars).[48] Depending upon whether they are manufactured for babies or toddlers, these items typically contain added sugar, a sugar source (such as corn syrup, dried cane syrup, or evaporated cane juice), fruit purée concentrates, and/or fruit juice concentrates as primary ingredients; these ingredients are all used to sweeten a product. When parents make a baby's food at home, these unnecessary sweeteners are avoided.

Preparing homemade baby food is easier and less time-consuming than many parents believe. And it is definitely more wholesome and less expensive than the baby foods that line the grocer's shelves. As a parent, you are given more control over your child's nutrition when you make your own baby food: You are guaranteed what is and is not going into your infant's food, what you are and are not adding to it, and that it is fresh rather than highly processed. In addition, there are more options as to what you can serve your baby because you are not limited to the types of baby foods sold in stores. Furthermore, you can customize the textures (such as thickness, lumpiness, or chunkiness) exactly to your baby's preferences and abilities.

Because it is fresh and has not been sitting on the shelf for weeks, foods prepared for your baby at home taste better than the baby foods available at the store. Better yet, when you serve fresh, wholesome foods to your little one, she learns to enjoy natural, unaltered flavors, which is critical in developing healthy eating habits early on. Moreover, unlike some commercial infant and toddler foods, you can be sure the foods you make your baby do not contain sugar, salt, starch, or any other additives.

Resources to help you prepare healthy, safe baby food from scratch abound. Cookbooks include *Top 100 Baby Purees, The Healthy Baby Meal Planner,* and *First Meals and More: Your Questions Answered* by Annabel Karmel; *Cooking for Baby: Wholesome, Homemade, Delicious Foods for Six to Eighteen Months* and *The Petit Appetit Cookbook* by Lisa Barnes; and *Homemade Baby Food Pure and Simple* by Connie Linardakis. A couple of helpful websites are WholesomeBabyFood.com and MyBabyFoodRecipes.com. However, making homemade baby food is not complicated. It can even be prepared in large batches and frozen in individual servings so that it does not require extra time and energy every day.

As a general guide, fruits and vegetables should be washed thoroughly, peeled and cored/pitted as necessary, chopped, and then steamed or boiled with a small amount of water until tender. Bananas and avocadoes, however, do not need to be cooked first. Simply purée them once they are peeled, or mash them well with a fork. Ensure that protein items (as age-appropriate) such as meat, poultry, fish, dried beans/peas/lentils, tofu, and egg yolk are cooked thoroughly. Once cooked, foods can be puréed using a food processor or blender. If any item is too thick or chunky, simply add water while puréeing. Spoon the puréed food into ice cube trays and freeze; once frozen, transfer the cubes into plastic freezer bags or containers and freeze for up to three months. Label freezer bags/containers with the date and contents, and pull out individual servings as needed each day. For food safety, thaw foods in the refrigerator rather than on the counter, and wash your hands, surfaces, equipment, and utensils with hot water and soap whenever you work with baby food. There is an exception: buying canned or frozen puréed pumpkin and butternut squash, cooking (if frozen), then freezing in individual servings is an acceptable alternative to preparing from scratch if you find that these are difficult or too time-consuming to prepare yourself. However, ensure that there are no other ingredients added to the products you purchase.

Keep in mind that infants only need baby food for a few months – not for their entire lives, so you will not have to specially prepare baby food forever. It is definitely worth the investment of time and energy early on to ensure that your infant gets off to the right start and that you set a solid foundation for the establishment of healthy eating habits.

Commercial Baby Foods

Mass-produced baby foods lack freshness because they are highly processed and then sit in the container for weeks or months before you feed them to your baby. Many contain ingredients and additives that are difficult to pronounce, which most parents desire to avoid when feeding their little one. In addition, manufactured baby foods lose valuable nutrients during processing. And last but not least, commercial baby foods are expensive.

Although baby food manufacturers market certain lines of baby foods such as "Stage 1®" and "1st Foods®" for babies less than six months of age, babies this young should not be eating solid foods yet. In fact, Project Viva found that formula-fed babies who begin eating solids before four months of age have a significantly greater risk of being obese at three years of age.[49] It is best to wait until an infant is closer to six months old to introduce solid baby foods.

The next few sections will address some specific food items manufactured for infants, toddlers, and preschoolers. It is necessary to preface this discussion with a disclaimer. First of all, every brand is not the same, so what may be true for one product may be entirely different than for a similar item distributed by another company. This is not intended to be an exhaustive list of all brands and varieties of foods produced for babies and young children, but merely to provide a snapshot. Furthermore, manufacturers' formulations change constantly, so what might be accurate information about a product today may be different tomorrow. Again, this is meant to be a general overview for the purpose of providing readers with an awareness of what is actually present in foods mass-produced for children. We will start by investigating a few popular categories of commercial baby food.

The cereal and fruit as well as the grain and fruit combinations manufactured for babies are high in sugar – although they are natural sugars, a baby's taste buds cannot distinguish the difference: sweet is sweet. These products contain fruit juice concentrates and/or fruit purée concentrates, which are equivalent in taste to sugar. Consumption of these sweet items is an unhealthy habit to begin during infancy, especially for breakfast or as a snack.

The same is true with some of the puréed fruit mixtures, particularly those that contain fruit purée concentrates and fruit juice concentrates. Although they do not contain any added sugars, some of these products taste like a dessert rather than fruit because of the high concentration of natural sugars.

Speaking of desserts, baby food desserts should not be manufactured in the first place because they contain large amounts of sugar and taste extremely sweet. The primary ingredients are fruit purée concentrates and/or fruit juice concentrates. Dessert items, including commercial baby food dessert products, should never be served to babies less than a year old.

Commercial Toddler and Preschooler Foods

Baby food companies have created an unnecessary industry, and this is especially true in regard to toddler and preschooler foods – stages when children no longer need puréed foods and their ability to chew and swallow various food textures becomes increasingly similar to those of the rest of the family. The meals, snacks, and other products that are being manufactured for toddlers and preschoolers are of great concern. Just as with baby foods, these items are highly processed; because of this, they lack freshness and contain preservatives and/or additives. Furthermore, they tend to be lower in essential nutrients, such as fiber, than their more fresh and wholesome counterparts. Even those touted as being made with whole grains contain very little, if any, fiber. However, there is even more at stake if we serve young children these mass-produced foods.

Sugar and Salt

The majority of items manufactured specifically for toddlers and preschoolers contain added sugar (and/or a sugar source, such as corn syrup, dried cane syrup, or evaporated cane juice) and/or salt, often as one of the first four ingredients.[50] In fact, many of the toddler and preschooler foods provide more than one-fourth of a young child's sodium needs for an entire day, while some provide nearly half of the daily sodium requirement.[51] Even the diced vegetables manufactured for toddlers contain added salt, while the diced fruits have fruit juice concentrate or fruit purée concentrate. Additions of these substances to otherwise nutrient-rich foods offer no nutritional benefits and can set youngsters up for a lifetime of unhealthy taste preferences.

Not only are large amounts of sugar and salt absolutely unnecessary and unhealthy for young ones' little bodies, but their taste buds, which are highly influenced during this time, become accustomed to these flavors early on; this will make it exceedingly difficult to convince kids to eat wholesome, nutritious foods in their future years.

Commercial Snacks for Infants, Toddlers, and Preschoolers

The majority of snacks manufactured for infants, toddlers, and preschoolers are of little or no nutritional value (refer to Table 1). Oftentimes they are so highly-sweetened that they may as well be a dessert. For example, cookies are not an appropriate snack for individuals of any age, much less infants and young children; cookies are to be reserved as a dessert item. More than that, cookies should not be served to infants in the first place, and offered only occasionally to toddlers and preschoolers. The cookies, including teething biscuits, marketed for infants and toddlers contain sugar and/or sources of sugar (high fructose corn syrup, evaporated cane juice, dried cane syrup, brown rice syrup), plus they provide no fiber. In addition, serving these treats to young ones teaches them the unhealthy habit of eating cookies and sweet items as a snack.

Certain brands of puffs – both fruit- and vegetable-flavored – offer no health benefits. The combination of sugar, fruit purée, and fruit juice concentrate (or sugar and a sweet vegetable purée) results in a sweet product, and they contain additives that infants and toddlers need not consume. Although they are made with a small amount of whole grains, they do not contain any fiber, and while they claim to be made with real fruit or vegetables, popular brands provide no vitamin A or C (an organic brand contains ten percent).

The cereal bars manufactured specifically for young children are high in sugar. In some cases, sugar is a primary ingredient, plus they contain additional sweetening agents like high fructose corn syrup and dextrose. A different variety contains evaporated cane juice and invert cane juice along with fruit juice concentrates and other sweeteners. Because they are highly processed, these bars also contain many additives. Even though they are marketed as being composed of whole grains, they contain less than one gram, if any, fiber; although touted to be made with real fruit, they contain no vitamin A or C (except for one type that contains a minimal amount of vitamin C).

The chewy fruit snacks contain a large amount of sugar yet provide very little nutrition. Depending upon the brand, they are mainly composed of fruit juice concentrates and fruit purée concentrates, sometimes in combination with sugar and corn syrup. These fruit chews are virtually like candy to a young child – certainly not a snack item. They also contain additives, such as carnauba wax and beeswax. While they may contain one hundred percent of a child's daily need for vitamin C, they essentially provide no other nutrients.

A child easily consumes plenty of vitamin C by eating alternative nutrient-rich foods, such as fresh fruit.

Yogurt-based bite-sized snacks contain sweeteners. In certain brands, sugar is the second ingredient, and the third ingredient is fruit purée. Some contain no whole grains and they all provide zero to less than one gram of fiber. On top of that, much processing and several additives are required to transform yogurt into an unrefrigerated finger food.

Table 1: Key Ingredients in Commercial Snacks for Young Children*

Type of Snack	Examples of Sweetening Agents**	Whole Grain Content	Fiber	Vitamin A	Vitamin C	Examples of Possible Additives**
Cookies	Sugar High Fructose Corn Syrup Corn Syrup Solids Fructose Dried Cane Syrup Brown Rice Syrup	Depends upon the brand and variety. For those that contain them, it is minimal.	0	0	0	Sodium acid pyrophosphate, Soy lecithin, Ammonium bicarbonate, Tricalcium phosphate, Mixed tocopherols (for freshness), DATEM, Whey (from milk), Natural butter flavor
Cinnamon Graham Crackers	Sugar High Fructose Corn Syrup Dried Cane Syrup	2 grams	0	0	0	Sodium acid pyrophosphate, Soy lecithin, Mixed tocopherols (for freshness), Whey (from milk), Natural flavor
Teething Biscuits	Sugar Evaporated Cane Juice	2 grams	0 to less than 1 gram	0	0	Ammonium bicarbonate, Soy lecithin, Tricalcium phosphate, Mixed tocopherols (for freshness), l-cysteine hydrochloride (dough conditioner), Natural butter flavor

Puffs	Sugar Fruit Purée Fruit Juice Concentrate	2 grams	0	0 to 10%	0 to 10%	Tri- and dicalcium phosphate, Mixed tocopherols (for freshness) , Soy lecithin, Sunflower lecithin, Caramel color, Turmeric extract color, Annatto extract color
Cereal Bars	Sugar High Fructose Corn Syrup Corn Syrup Dextrose Evaporated Cane Juice Invert Cane Juice Fruit Juice Concentrates Fruit Powder Honey	2 grams	0 to less than 1 gram	0	0 (One type contains 6%)	Glycerin, Modified cornstarch, Cellulose gel, Xanthan gum, Cellulose gum, Pectin, Locust bean gum, Tapioca starch, Carageenan gum, Wheat gluten, Annatto (for color)
Chewy Fruit Snacks	Fruit Juice Concentrates Fruit Purée Concentrates Sugar Corn Syrup Dextrose	0	0	0	100%	Carnauba wax, Beeswax Carageenan, Pectin, Hydrogenated coconut oil, Cornstarch, Citrus fiber, Paprika extract color, Natural flavor
Yogurt-Based Bite-Sized Snacks	Sugar Fruit Purée Fruit Juice Concentrate Cane Juice Powder (evaporated cane juice, invert cane juice) Fruit Powder	Depends upon the brand.	0 to less than 1 gram	0 to 15%	0 to 10%	Tapioca starch, Gelatin, Lactic acid esters of mono- and diglycerides, Dicalcium phosphate, Annatto extract color, Soy lecithin, Natural flavor

Snack ingredients, formulations, and nutrition information may change. Please refer to current product packaging for the most accurate and up-to-date nutrition facts.

**Products do not contain all of the sweeteners or additives listed. This table provides a conglomeration of examples from several products and brands.*

Commercial Beverages for Infants, Toddlers, and Preschoolers

To begin with, there is no need for infants or young children to ingest sweetened yogurt, whether it is manufactured by a baby food company or mainstream brand. These products are high in sugar and taste sweet. Instead, youngsters can be served plain yogurt (or cottage cheese), which they will readily accept if they have not become accustomed to sweetened flavors. Yogurt juice is even more concerning. When fruit purée concentrates and fruit juice concentrates are combined with yogurt, the result is an extremely sweet product that contains significantly more sugar and calories than one hundred percent fruit juice.

Furthermore, the dairy beverages marketed for toddlers and preschoolers are completely unnecessary. First of all, they contain flavoring and/or sweeteners. Secondly, a child can drink plain unsweetened milk, whether it is cow's milk or an alternative due to a milk allergy or intolerance. And last, these flavored beverages contain additives that are not necessary in regular milk.

The water and fruit juice blends for toddlers and preschoolers are addressed earlier in this chapter in "The Truth about Juice" section. These drinks are basically fruit juice concentrates diluted with water. Although they contain fewer calories and sugar than one hundred percent fruit juice (because extra water is added), they are still flavorful. The bottom line is that young children need to become accustomed to drinking plain water, not sweetened or otherwise-flavored water. The fruit juices manufactured by the baby food companies are also discussed in "The Truth about Juice" section of this chapter; to reiterate, there is nothing special about these products and young children, especially babies, do not need to drink fruit juice in the first place.

Commercial Baby Foods are Convenience Items

Commercial baby, toddler, and preschooler meals and foods are actually convenience items; that is, they are to be used occasionally, for the sake of convenience. Some examples include: when there is no refrigeration available, when you are taking your baby on an airplane, or when your family is taking a long road trip. And if used in that way, manufactured baby foods are not harmful or unhealthy for young ones. However, Americans have fallen into the trap of regularly feeding our infants and toddlers these mass-produced foods, which is a contributing factor to the widespread problem of poor diet and health among children in our country.

Although convenient, a steady diet of processed foods pollutes children's bodies over time, especially if introduced in their formative years. Adults are aware that we should not regularly eat processed foods; thus, it stands to reason that we need to be even more vigilant about how often kids – and to a greater extent, infants, toddlers, and preschoolers – consume such items. Unfortunately, we feed these products to our young children daily, often without realizing that they are highly processed and unwholesome. Parents know that it is unhealthy for families to routinely consume meals out of a can, box, freezer, or microwave. In the same way, it is inappropriate for babies, toddlers, and preschoolers to eat items that originate in a jar or package on a regular basis. Not only is it unhealthy for their growing bodies, it is not a habit that we want them to develop, especially at such an impressionable age.

Baby and toddler foods manufactured by the baby food companies do not need to be banned altogether. But as described previously, they should only be used occasionally – in "emergency" type situations – when there really are no other options and convenience is more important than health, which is rare. Because preschoolers can virtually eat the same foods that the rest of the family eats, there is actually no need for preschooler meals or snacks, even on an occasional basis.

When selecting manufactured baby and toddler foods for those occasional instances, the healthiest choices should be made; for example, cookies should not be purchased as a snack option. Here is a parallel: fast-food will not cause us to become overweight and unhealthy if it is only eaten occasionally and if good choices are made when it is eaten. In the same way, commercial baby and toddler foods will not cause our children to become unhealthy or to establish poor eating habits if these products are consumed once in a great while, and if the best options are chosen for those times. Wise choices include items that contain the least amounts of sugar/sweeteners, sodium/salt, additives, and preservatives. The most nutritious selections are those that are also good sources of whole grains, fiber, vitamins, and minerals. Additionally, search for products that are minimally processed. In general, the closer a food is to its natural state, the less processed it is.

Healthy and Appropriate Meal and Snack Options

Healthy eating recommendations for toddlers and preschoolers include: increasing consumption of fruits and vegetables to at least five servings per day, eating more fiber-rich grains, switching from high-fat dairy products to low-fat (1%) or fat-free (skim) dairy products after the age of two, and eating family meals that are prepared at home.[52] A simple way to gauge your child's daily nutritional intake is to ask yourself questions like, "How many times did my child consume fresh fruit today?" and, "Did he or she eat any vegetables?"

Although it depends upon a child's age as well as his developmental abilities, there are plenty of healthy, affordable meal and snack alternatives to those that are mass-produced for infants and young children.

- Plain single-grain baby cereals: rice, brown rice, barley, or oatmeal with no fruit or other sweetening agents added. Plain multi-grain baby cereal is appropriate for older babies who tolerate single-grain cereals.

- Unsweetened whole grain dry cereals such as Original Cheerios®, Corn and Rice Chex®, Original Wheaties®, and Original Whole Grain Total®. More dense cereals like Wheat Chex®, Quaker® Crunchy Corn Bran, and Original Bite-Sized Shredded Wheat (soaked in milk) are appropriate for older toddlers and preschoolers.

- Pieces of one hundred percent whole wheat (or other one hundred percent whole grain) toast, bread, pita bread, bagels (miniature bagels are the perfect size and a favorite of youngsters), and tortillas

- Soft-cooked whole grain pasta, mashed or chopped into small pieces

- Small pieces of natural cheese; plain yogurt; plain cottage cheese

- Fresh bananas and avocadoes, mashed or chopped

- Unsweetened natural applesauce

- Fruits and vegetables – soft-cooked and puréed or mashed for infants; peeled and/or cooked as necessary and diced into small pieces or shredded for toddlers; "harder" fruits and vegetables, such as apples, melon, and carrots, need to be soft-cooked and then diced for younger toddlers until these foods are no longer a choking hazard.

- Raisins, dried cranberries, and other small pieces of dried fruit for older toddlers and preschoolers, in small amounts because they are a concentrated source of sugar and taste really sweet. (These are a choking hazard for infants and young toddlers.)

- Freeze-dried miniature fruit snacks manufactured for toddlers, in moderation. Although sweet, they are one hundred percent fruit and contain no additives or other ingredients. However, these provide very few nutrients, so offer occasionally and sparingly.

- Protein – tender lean meats and poultry; freshly-prepared soft fish with bones removed; tofu; dried beans, peas, and lentils; egg (no egg white until at least one year of age): puréed, mashed, or soft-cooked and chopped into small pieces

- In addition to these suggestions, older toddlers and preschoolers can basically eat what the rest of the family is eating (assuming the family is consuming nutritious meals and snacks), with the appropriate texture modifications, of course; these little ones definitely do not require already-prepared meals and snacks out of a package.

In summary, a primary concern about exposing infants, toddlers, and preschoolers to sweet and salty foods is that these impressionable youngsters are practically becoming addicted to these flavors at a young age. Commercial baby, toddler, and preschooler foods serve to fuel that addiction. We cannot expect children to develop a palate for unsweetened, low-sodium, naturally-flavored foods if we feed them highly-flavorful sweet or salty products starting in the early days of their life. Raising young children on a steady diet of sweet, salty, savory foods guarantees that they will desire and demand these types of foods as they grow up.

On the other hand, foods that are made fresh at home are less processed and more wholesome than those purchased off of the grocer's shelves. Because of this, homemade foods are more likely to provide valuable nutrients, such as fiber and cancer-fighting phytochemicals, yet contain less sugar, sodium, additives, and preservatives.

Please keep in mind that while it is never too early to teach children healthy eating habits, it is also never too late. Do not despair if your teenager's daily diet consists of zero vegetables, little fruit, and predominantly junk food. There is hope. It may not be as easy to improve his eating pattern as if he was two years old, but it is possible to change his dietary habits, and it will be well worth it. The next chapter describes just one step that can be taken in that direction: a healthy breakfast.

5 A HEALTHY BREAKFAST

Jada, a teenager, skips breakfast every weekday morning for a variety of reasons. Foremost, Jada is trying to lose weight, and she believes that skipping a meal will help her achieve this goal. Besides that, she lacks the time to eat something before heading out the door to school in the morning. Additionally, Jada's parents do not consume anything more substantial than coffee before noon, so she is merely imitating what she has observed. Jada's final reason, quite simply, is that there are no healthy breakfast foods available in her home. Unfortunately, Jada is suffering the consequences of skipping the most important meal of the day. First of all, Jada is excessively tired and lacks energy at school in the morning. Next, she continues to gain weight rather than lose it. This is largely because she is famished by the time she gets home from school, even if she eats something for lunch, so she overeats. Making matters worse, she often grabs unhealthy, high-calorie snack foods in order to quickly ease her hunger. Lastly, she is performing poorly in school because she is unable to focus or concentrate. But because Jada does not understand the importance of eating breakfast, she does not realize the connection between skipping it and the negative outcomes she is experiencing.

Americans are familiar with the adage, "Breakfast is the most important meal of the day." However, this well-known saying omits a key message: a *healthy* breakfast is the most important meal of the day. While regularly missing any meal can have adverse effects on an individual's weight and health status, breakfast is particularly essential, especially for growing children and adolescents. As the first meal after a night of fasting, breakfast gives the body the energy it needs to start the day; it also provides the brain with the fuel it requires to function. These two benefits of eating a healthy breakfast are critical for kids as they sit in school classrooms to learn, where they need to perform well academically and exhibit appropriate behavior and self-control.

The Increase in Breakfast-Skipping

Over the same period of time, both obesity and breakfast-skipping have become increasingly prevalent in America, despite increased knowledge about the importance of a healthy breakfast.[1,2] For instance, between the mid-sixties and early-nineties, the number of adults who missed breakfast rose from less than fifteen percent to twenty-five percent.[3,4] And kids have followed their example: breakfast intake by children and adolescents has declined over time, most significantly among older children and adolescents. Over the course of about two-and-half decades, breakfast consumption fell by five percent in preschoolers, almost ten percent among eight to ten year olds, and up to twenty percent among adolescents.[5]

Children and adolescents skip breakfast more than any other meal, with the frequency increasing as they get older.[6] Data from the National Heart, Lung, and Blood Institute (NHLBI) Growth and Healthy Study reveals that two to seventeen percent of young children skip breakfast, while fifteen to nineteen percent of adolescents miss breakfast.[7] Another analysis found that more than twenty percent of eight to nine year olds and over forty percent of twelve to thirteen year olds report that they do not eat breakfast on a daily basis.[8] Researchers also discovered that nearly sixty percent – well over half – of high school students skip breakfast more than three times a week.

In regards to adolescent females, approximately eighty-four percent ate breakfast in the mid-sixties whereas by the early-nineties, only about sixty-five percent reported eating breakfast.[9] Furthermore, approximately one in four skip breakfast on any given day, and less than thirty percent report eating breakfast every day. In addition, about one-third of female teenagers between fifteen and eighteen years of age skip breakfast on a regular basis.[10] Breakfast consumption has also declined among male adolescents, from almost ninety percent in the mid-sixties to seventy-five percent in the early-nineties.[11] These trends are a serious concern because eating habits established during adolescence, along with the risk of chronic disease associated with those patterns, tend to persist into adulthood.[12] Thus, the time to address nutrition issues such as skipping meals/breakfast is during childhood, before they reach adolescence.

In my professional experience of providing nutrition counseling to patients, breakfast is the meal that is most often skipped or insufficient in quantity and quality; it is often eaten quickly while on-the-go to school or work and composed of items low in fiber and high in sugar. It is not uncommon for individuals who do not consume three well-rounded meals each day – whether they skip breakfast, lunch, and/or dinner – to compensate for that missed or inadequate meal by overeating later that day or night. This type of erratic eating pattern results in a poor nutritional intake as well as unwanted weight gain.

Parental Influence on Breakfast Habits

It is imperative that adults, specifically parents and caregivers, encourage children and adolescents to eat a healthy breakfast while at the same time explaining the advantages of doing so. Ideally, this would start in early childhood and continue through adolescence; it is especially crucial among those who are most likely to skip it, such as older children and adolescents – particularly teenage girls. More than that, parents have a responsibility to plan, promote, prepare, and provide wholesome, balanced breakfast foods for their children. Perhaps most importantly, parents can serve as role models for their children by eating a healthy breakfast every morning. In fact, parental breakfast habits have been found to be a significant indicator of adolescent breakfast habits.[13]

The perceptions that children and adolescents develop regarding breakfast may effect whether or not they eat it. For example, females frequently avoid breakfast because they believe it will cause them to gain weight.[14,15] On the other hand, many children feel that breakfast gives them energy and improves their ability to pay attention at school.[16] Parents must be mindful of their own influence and diligently work at helping children shape their beliefs and attitudes about breakfast – and to correct any misconceptions children might have about this all-important meal.

Benefits of a Healthy Breakfast

Skipping breakfast has been linked with several negative consequences. Conversely, research shows that children and adolescents who routinely consume a nourishing breakfast benefit both nutritionally and academically. In fact, some experts believe that a nutritious breakfast is essential for optimizing health and preventing chronic disease among children and adolescents.[17]

Nutrition Status

A healthy breakfast improves a child's nutritional intake and overall dietary quality. Consistently eating breakfast is associated with higher nutrient intakes, more nutritious food choices, and regular eating habits, as well as healthy habits like physical activity.[18,19] On the other hand, children and adolescents who do not eat breakfast are apt to have diets that are considered poor or inadequate; skipping breakfast leads to nutritional inadequacies that are not made up for at meals or snacks during the rest of the day.[20]

According to research, children and adolescents who regularly eat breakfast have higher nutrient intakes and are more likely to consume an adequate amount of nutrients than those who skip breakfast.[21,22] By eating breakfast, children and adolescents obtain a greater amount of essential nutrients, vitamins, and minerals, including protein, fiber, folic acid, and calcium.[23,24] This is significant because the diets of many children and adolescents lack important nutrients, such as fiber; vitamin A; B vitamins, including folic acid; as well as minerals like calcium, iron, and zinc.[25,26] In some cases the gap is substantial and disconcerting. Interestingly, these nutrients are typically consumed as part of a nutritious, well-balanced breakfast. Moreover, breakfast eaters usually have lower-fat diets and lower cholesterol levels than those who regularly miss breakfast.[27,28]

Those who eat breakfast also tend to eat healthier throughout the course of a day compared to those who do not. For instance, breakfast eaters consume more vegetables and milk, less soda, and fewer French fries.[29] Part of this is due to the fact that a morning meal reduces impulsive snacking while preventing erratic eating patterns and overeating later in the day – which is when high-calorie, high-fat, high-sugar, and/or high-salt foods are usually chosen. Likewise, high-fiber cereal with milk is a common breakfast choice; this type of meal provides long-lasting satiety and prevents hunger.

Weight Status

Contrary to popular belief, skipping breakfast is not a good method for weight loss or weight management. A study conducted among individuals in the National Weight Control Registry proves that the majority of adults who are able to maintain substantial weight loss long-term routinely eat a healthy breakfast.[30] What is more, an inverse correlation has been observed between breakfast consumption and body mass index (BMI): Breakfast eaters typically have healthier BMIs than those who miss it, and those who skip or eat an unsubstantial morning meal are more likely to be obese with a high BMI.[31] This reverse relationship remains significant even after adjusting for other possible causes, including gender, age, race, socioeconomic status, and lifestyle factors. As discussed in chapter one, a normal/healthy BMI is associated with a healthy body weight while a high BMI may indicate overweight or obesity.

Children and adolescents who habitually skip or eat an inadequate breakfast have significantly greater risk of being overweight or obese. Research reveals that children and adolescents who miss breakfast have higher body weights or BMIs than those who normally consume a morning meal. For example, a study found that eating breakfast on a regular basis decreases the likelihood of obesity among girls and overweight/obesity among boys by about thirty percent.[32] Similarly, girls who normally eat breakfast tend to have lower BMIs than girls who skip it.[33,34] One analysis reports that children who do not typically eat breakfast have nearly double the chance of being overweight compared to those who usually do eat it.[35] Further, adolescents who consistently eat breakfast often have lower BMIs than teenagers who regularly skip it.[36,37] In addition, overweight and obese children and adolescents miss breakfast much more frequently than their normal-weight counterparts.[38,39]

Possibly most convincing is that a healthy breakfast appears to reduce the occurrence of overweight and obesity even among youths who are at high-risk: Adolescents who have at least one obese parent and consume breakfast on a daily basis tend to have healthier BMIs than those who do not eat breakfast.[40] And low-income girls who take part in a School Breakfast, School Lunch, and/or Food Stamp Program dramatically reduce their probability of being overweight.[41] This is significant because it proves that breakfast acts as a safeguard and preventative measure in the fight against obesity, not only in general, but even amongst kids who are most susceptible to developing the condition. Therefore, whether your child is at low-risk or high-risk, ensuring a nutritious daily breakfast is crucial for providing protection against obesity.

The Relationship between Skipping Breakfast and Unhealthy Snacking

As breakfast-skipping has become more common over the years, the prevalence of snacking and the amounts of calories and nutrients derived from snack foods have also increased.[42] In fact, missing breakfast has been linked to a greater occurrence of snacking and the consumption of high-fat snacks.[43] As mentioned earlier, this is likely due to the fact that missing the critical morning meal, typically composed of vital nutrient-rich foods, leads to extreme hunger and unhealthy snacking. Adding to the problem is that the snack foods typically consumed by youth are often high in calories, fat, sugar, and/or salt, as well as low in vitamins and minerals; for instance, soda is one of the most common snacks among adolescent females.[44]

Cognitive Function and Academic Performance

Again and again, research confirms that breakfast boosts brain power. First of all, breakfast prevents morning-time hunger; hunger itself is known to contribute to emotional, behavioral, and academic problems among both children and adolescents.[45] More than that, multiple studies report that breakfast enhances a child's cognitive function and ability to learn at school.[46,47] For example, students who eat a well-balanced breakfast earn better grades and higher test scores than those who do not; children who eat breakfast also demonstrate improved memory.[48] Some of the greatest gains appear to be made in mathematics, a subject that requires intense concentration and attention to detail.[49,50]

However, the advantages of a healthy breakfast extend past a boost in mental abilities. Research reveals that breakfast leads to better school attendance and lower rates of tardiness.[51,52] In addition, eating a good breakfast has been noted to improve classroom behavior and attentiveness, as well as result in fewer discipline problems at school.[53,54] Moreover, students who eat breakfast make fewer visits to the school office and the school nurse.[55] Beyond that, both parents and children report marked improvement in psychosocial function when children regularly eat an adequate breakfast: Studies show that breakfast consumption has a positive effect on symptoms of depression and hyperactivity.[56] In the same way, a wholesome breakfast has been found to enhance mood, including levels of alertness and contentment.

Benefits of Breakfast Cereal

One of the best and most convenient choices for a nourishing breakfast is unsweetened, low-fat whole grain hot or cold cereal. In fact, the majority of cereal eaten in the United States is consumed at breakfast, and cereal is a major source of essential nutrients for children and adolescents in America.[57,58] Multiple studies reveal that not only is eating breakfast beneficial, but more specifically, that there are advantages of having cereal for breakfast. This has led researchers to conclude that the positive effects of a wholesome breakfast may be enhanced if cereal is part of the meal.[59] The advantages of cereal consumption in particular are likely related to the facts that cereals are typically fortified with multiple vitamins and minerals, often low in fat and cholesterol, usually a good source of fiber, and frequently consumed with nutrient-rich milk.[60,61]

Cereal is a significant source of several important nutrients, especially for children and adolescents. Both the NHLBI Growth and Health Study and a National Health and Nutrition Examination Survey (NHANES) found that the daily intake of key nutrients such as protein, fiber, vitamin A, vitamin C, B vitamins (including folic acid), calcium, iron, and zinc are considerably higher among those who eat cereal for breakfast.[62,63] Further, those that eat cereal for their morning meal have notably lower fat and cholesterol intakes.[64,65] Additionally, cereal is an excellent source of whole grains. Whole grains are a vital part of the diet and provide numerous health benefits; packed with fiber, antioxidants, and phytochemicals, whole grains aid in reducing the risk of obesity, heart disease, stroke, diabetes, and cancer.

Research also shows that individuals who frequently eat cereal for breakfast are less likely to be overweight or obese. One study demonstrates that children who frequently eat cereal have healthier BMIs and lower risk of overweight and obesity than those who eat cereal less often.[66] Cereal consumption has also been associated with lower BMIs and decreased chance of overweight and obesity among adolescents and young adults.[67] According to data from NHANES, adults who have hot or cold cereal for breakfast have lower BMIs compared to those who skip or consume a less-nutritious breakfast, like meat and eggs.[68] What is more, children and adolescents who routinely eat cereal have lower cholesterol levels than those who rarely or never have cereal.[69]

Breakfast Recommendations

The following recommendations are based upon suggestions from the authors of a thorough article, "Breakfast Habits, Nutritional Status, Body Weight, and Academic Performance in Children and Adolescents," published in the *Journal of the American Dietetic Association*.[70] These researchers concluded that there is strong evidence indicating that a healthy breakfast improves the overall health and well-being of children and adolescents, and that the advantages of breakfast appear to affect individuals of all ages, demographic groups, and socioeconomic levels.

- Children and adolescents need to eat a healthy breakfast every day – either at home, at school, or on the way to school.

- Include a variety of foods, such as whole grains, fruit, and low-fat dairy, for a well-balanced breakfast. Unsweetened, low-fat whole grain cereals that are fortified with vitamins and minerals and rich in fiber appear to offer nutritional advantages, particularly when paired with low-fat milk.

- Choose low-fat dairy products, and on occasion lean breakfast meats, in order to reduce total fat and saturated fat consumption. However, toddlers between one and two years of age need to consume whole milk for brain development.

- Children and adolescents who skip breakfast because they do not have time can be encouraged to wake up earlier or eat breakfast on the way to school or at school. When you think creatively, there are a variety of healthy, wholesome breakfast items that can be eaten on-the-go: a whole grain bagel or toast; unsweetened, dry whole grain cereal in a plastic bag or container, mixed with dried fruit and/or unsalted nuts, if desired; a low-fat, lower-sugar whole grain granola bar, breakfast bar, or muffin; low-fat yogurt topped with unsweetened whole grain cereal; fresh fruit; a hard-boiled egg; a fruit smoothie made with fresh and/or unsweetened frozen fruit and low-fat milk or yogurt; a single serving of low-fat milk in a portable container (one hundred percent fruit juice is acceptable occasionally, such as once a week). For a complete and filling breakfast, mix and match two to three of these options, for example: a one hundred percent whole wheat bagel, grapes, and a hard-boiled egg; or a healthy granola bar, a banana, and low-fat milk.

- Alternative calcium sources, such as calcium-fortified milk alternatives (like soy or rice milk), one hundred percent juice, or other calcium-rich foods, should be consumed by those who cannot or will not consume milk or dairy products; an inadequate intake of dairy can result in a low intake of other nutrients, including protein and vitamins A and D. If this is an issue with your child, consider scheduling an appointment with a registered dietitian to ensure he is getting an adequate amount of nutrients. Lactose-free milks are available for children with lactose intolerance.

- If available and appropriate, take advantage of the School Breakfast Program at your child's school. Ensure that healthy options are selected.

Breakfast Cereals

It is critical to be astute when selecting breakfast cereals – both hot and cold varieties. Begin by studying the nutrition facts panel. Opt for those that are: unsweetened and low in sugar, with less than eight grams of sugar per serving; low in fat, containing no more than three to four grams of fat; composed primarily – if not entirely – of whole grains, such as one hundred percent whole wheat or one hundred percent whole grain oats; and a good source of fiber, with at least three to five grams of fiber serving. Bear in mind that children and adolescents rarely consume only one serving of cereal, which is generally three-quarters cup to one cup. It is not uncommon for children to eat at least two to three servings at a time, so usually more than one serving's worth of sugar and fat is ingested.

It is alarming to walk down the cereal aisle at the grocery store. Nearly every week, at least one new type of sugar-coated cereal appears on the shelves. Not only are these highly-sweetened so-called breakfast products unhealthy for kids in the short-term, but they can also have negative long-term effects as well. For example, a major concern is that their sweet flavor could contribute to the development of a preference for sugary foods, notably sweetened breakfast items.[71] Because of this, if a certain cereal contains less than eight grams of sugar but is in some way sweetened or tastes sweet to you, do not serve it to your child for breakfast.

The marketing strategies for sweetened cereals have always been very effective. No one could ever forget a little leprechaun singing, "They're magically delicious!" or Tony the Tiger™

exclaiming, "They're Gr-r-reat!®" And who could outgrow memories of Toucan Sam™, that "silly rabbit," or the cute honey bee? Nowadays it appears that Honey Nut Cheerios® is one of the least adulterated options in the cereal aisle. The sugar-laden choices have become widespread, and it can be difficult to find the unsweetened, more wholesome options on the shelves. Take, for example, Eggo® Maple Syrup cereal, Smorz® cereal, Reese's Puffs®, Rice Krispies Treats® cereal, Marshmallow Pebbles®, Sprinkles Cookie Crisp®, or Cocoa Puffs® Brownie Crunch. It is a wonderland for children – Disneyland® at the supermarket! Making matters worse is that these sugary cereals are located on the lowest shelves, directly within a child's eyesight and reach, while the low-sugar, high-fiber brands are up on the top shelves, almost out of an adult's reach. This is done very purposefully. Sales and marketing departments know that parents typically purchase the products that their children ask – or beg – for, and so these tempting products are intentionally placed in a child's plain view and grasp.

Every adult – parents and grandparents, teachers and coaches, doctors and nurses – must become voices of reason and advocates for children. No one else will speak up to them or for them. And if we neglect this responsibility, kids will not know any better. They are inundated. We have all seen (and can recite) the advertising campaigns on television; we have strolled down the cereal aisle and observed the bright, fun cereal boxes situated down at a youngster's level. The breakfast companies' marketing strategies are brilliant. We have to fight back. And that involves more than insisting that the television commercials aimed at youth be regulated or limited.

That is only part of the picture, albeit a large part. There is more to consider: packaging, websites, promotions, toy and game offers, cartoon characters, and so on. Simply browse some of the specific cereal websites geared towards children and adolescents, such as Kellogg's Frosted Flakes® at FrostedFlakes.com, Reese's Puffs® at ReesesPuffs.com, or Post® Pebbles® cereals at PebblesPlay.com. These businesses know what it takes to get the attention of kids and teenagers, and it is working.

Breakfast Cereal or Milk and Cookies?

Breakfast companies are basically manufacturing and promoting the equivalent of cookies disguised as breakfast cereals. And in some cases, this is not a metaphor – the cereal is literally composed of cookies! Would you allow your child to sit down to a plate of cookies and a glass of milk before sending her off to school? For the majority of parents and guardians, the idea is absurd. However, when we serve a bowl of sweetened cereal to a child, we are essentially feeding her milk and cookies for breakfast.

Please refer to Tables 1 and 2, which indicate the sugar and fiber content of certain sweetened cereals (Table 1) and selected cookies (Table 2). Notice that there are no significant differences between the various brands of cereals and cookies, and it is not uncommon for a serving of cookies to actually contain less sugar and/or more fiber than a serving of sweetened cereal. For example, with ten grams of sugar and two grams of fiber, a serving of one hundred percent Whole Grain Chips Ahoy® cookies (three cookies) provides less sugar and more fiber than three-fourths of a cup of several sweetened cereals, including Kellogg's Frosted Flakes®,

Cap'n Crunch's Crunch Berries®, and Cocoa Pebbles®. It is true
that breakfast cereals typically contain more vitamins and minerals
than cookies, however, most of these nutrients are not naturally-
occurring and have been added to the cereal during processing.
When it comes down to it, sweetened breakfast cereals – although
tasty and sometimes boasting specific nutrients – are contaminating
children's bodies and minds. Excess amounts of sugar first thing in
the morning do not benefit children nutritionally or academically,
and are likely to have an undesirable impact. More than that, they
are establishing a lifelong habit that, over time, may erode their
health and well-being, if not their teeth.

**TABLE 1: Comparison of Sugar and Fiber Content of Selected
Sweetened Cereals***

Cereal	Sugar per Serving (g)	Fiber per Serving (g)
Kellogg's'		
Frosted Flakes, Reduced Sugar with Fiber (per ¾ cup)	8	3
Corn Pops® (per 1 cup serving)	10	3
Frosted Flakes (per ¾ cup serving)	11	Less than 1
Cinnabon® Cereal (per 1 cup serving)	12	1
Eggo® Maple Syrup Cereal (per 1 cup serving)	12	2
Froot Loops® (per 1 cup serving) Apple Jacks® (per 1 cup serving)	12	3
Smorz® (per 1 cup serving)	13	Less than 1
Froot Loops® Marshmallow (per 1 cup serving)	14	2
Honey Smacks® (per ¾ cup serving)	15	1
General Mills		
Cookie Crisp® (per ¾ cup serving) Sprinkles Cookie Crisp® (per ¾ cup serving) Frosted Toast Crunch™ (per ¾ cup serving)	9	1
Cocoa Puffs® Brownie Crunch (per ¾ cup serving)	9	2

Trix® (per 1 cup serving) Chocolate Lucky Charms® (per ¾ cup serving) Reese's Puffs® (per ¾ cup serving) Count Chocula® (per ¾ cup serving) Frankenberry® (per 1 cup serving) Boo Berry® (per 1 cup serving)	10	1
Cinnamon Toast Crunch® (per ¾ cup serving) Golden Grahams® (per ¾ cup serving) Lucky Charms® (per ¾ cup serving) Cocoa Puffs® (per ¾ cup serving)	10	2
Quaker*		
Cap'n Crunch's Peanut Butter Crunch® (per ¾ cup serv)	9	1
Cap'n Crunch's Crunch Berries® (per ¾ cup serving) Cap'n Crunch's Chocolatey Crunch® (per ¾ cup serving)	11	1
Cap'n Crunch® Original (per ¾ cup serving) Honey Graham Oh's® (per ¾ cup serving)	12	1
Cap'n Crunch's OOPS! All Berries® (per 1 cup serving)	15	1
Post*		
Marshmallow Pebbles® (per ¾ cup serving)	10	0
Honeycomb® (per 1½ cup serving)	10	1
Alpha-Bits® (per 1 cup serving)	10	2
Fruity Pebbles® (per ¾ cup serving) Cocoa Pebbles® (per ¾ cup serving)	11	0
Waffle Crisp® (per 1 cup serving)	12	Less than 1
Golden Crisp® (per ¾ cup serving)	14	Less than 1

* *Cereal ingredients, formulations, and nutrition information may change. Please refer to current product packaging for the most accurate and up-to-date nutrition facts.*

TABLE 2: Comparison of Sugar and Fiber Content of Selected Cookie Varieties*

Cookie	Sugar (Grams)	Fiber (Grams)
Nabisco* Chips Ahoy* Cookies		
Chunky Chocolate Chunk (1 cookie)	5	0
Chunky White Fudge (1 cookie)	6	0
Chewy Chocolate Chip and Oatmeal (2 cookies)	8	1

With Reese's® Peanut Butter Cups (2 cookies) With Heath® English Toffee Bars (2 cookies)	9	1
Chewy Chocolate Chip (2 cookies)	10	1
100% Whole Grain Chocolate Chip (3 cookies)	10	2
Original Chocolate Chip (3 cookies)	11	1
Chewy Gooey Chocofudge (2 cookies) Chewy Gooey Megafudge (2 cookies)	13	1
Nabisco' Cookies		
Lorna Doone® Shortbread (4 cookies)	6	0
Nutter Butter' Sandwich Cookies (2 cookies)	8	1
Cameo® Crème Sandwich Cookies (2 cookies)	10	0
Oreo® Golden Original Sandwich Cookies (3 cookies)	12	0
Oreo® Chocolate Sandwich Cookies (3 cookies)	14	1
Nilla® Wafers (8 cookies) Ginger Snaps® (4 cookies)	11	0
Keebler' Animal Cookies		
Original Animal Crackers (8 crackers)	7	Less than 1
Iced (6 cookies)	8	Less than 1
Frosted (8 cookies)	13	Less than 1
Keebler' Cookies		
Sandies' Simply Shortbread (2 cookies)	7	0
Sandies' Pecan Shortbread (2 cookies)	7	Less than 1
Sandies' Chocolate Chip & Pecan Shortbread (2 cookies)	8	Less than 1
Vanilla Wafers (8 cookies) Chips Deluxe® Original (2 cookies) Chips Deluxe® Soft 'n Chewy (2 cookies) Fudge Shoppe® Peanut Butter Filled (2 cookies)	9	Less than 1
Fudge Shoppe® Fudge Stripes⁻ (3 cookies) Fudge Shoppe® Deluxe Grahams (3 cookies) Vienna Fingers® Crème Filled (2 cookies)	10	Less than 1
Chips Deluxe® Oatmeal Chocolate Chip (2 cookies)	10	1
Fudge Shoppe® Grasshopper® (4 cookies)	12	Less than 1
E.L. Fudge® Original (2 cookies)	12	1
E.L. Fudge® Double Stuffed (2 cookies)	13	1
Pepperidge Farm' Cookies		

Dark Chocolate Nantucket˜ Cookies (1 cookie) Homestyle Lemon Cookies (4 cookies)	8	0
Orange Milano® Cookies (2 cookies) Raspberry Milano® Cookies (2 cookies)	8	Less than 1
Verona® Strawberry Cookies (3 cookies) Soft Baked Sanibel® Snickerdoodle (1 cookie)	9	Less than 1
Sausalito˜ Milk Chocolate Macadamia (1 cookie) Soft Baked Mantauk˜ Milk Chocolate (1 cookie)	10	0
Homestyle Coconut Cookies (4 cookies)	10	2
Original Milano® Cookies (3 cookies) Homestyle Sugar Cookies (3 cookies)	11	Less than 1
Milk Chocolate Milano® Cookies (3 cookies)	13	Less than 1
Soft Baked Santa Cruz˜ Oatmeal Raisin (1 cookie)	13	2
Grandma's˜ Cookies		
Homestyle Peanut Butter Big Cookie (1 cookie)	10	2
Homestyle Chocolate Chip Big Cookie (1 cookie)	11	Less than 1
Peanut Butter Sandwich Crème (5 cookies)	11	2
Vanilla Sandwich Crème Cookies (5 cookies)	12	Less than 1
Homestyle Oatmeal Raisin Big Cookie (1 cookie)	12	2
Homestyle Peanut Butter Chocolate Chunks (1 cookie)	12	3
Mother's˜ Cookies		
Oatmeal (2 cookies)	8	Less than 1
Macaroons (2 cookies)	8	1
Coconut Cocadas® (5 cookies) Iced Lemonade (4 cookies)	9	Less than 1
Vanilla Crème Sandwich Cookies (2 cookies)	11	Less than 1
Original Frosted Circus Animals˜ (6 cookies) English Tea˜ (2 cookies)	12	Less than 1
Peanut Butter Gauchos® (2 cookies)	12	1
Double Fudge Sandwich Cookies (2 cookies)	13	1
Taffy˜ Sandwich Cookies (2 cookies)	16	Less than 1

Cookie ingredients, formulations, and nutrition information may change. Please refer to current product packaging for the most accurate and up-to-date nutrition facts.

As noted earlier, individuals typically eat more than one serving of cereal at a sitting because a serving size is so small. Therefore, when analyzing the nutrition facts label on a cereal box, it is probably necessary to double, triple, or even quadruple the amount of sugar listed in order to determine the actual amount of sugar consumed. So taking Froot Loops® or Waffle Crisp® as examples (refer to Table 2), your child probably ingests more than twelve grams of sugar when he eats that cereal. He could be consuming as much as thirty-six to forty-eight grams of sugar, equivalent to approximately three to four tablespoons (note: that is tablespoons, not teaspoons) of sugar; to picture this amount in your head, visualize nine to twelve cubes of sugar. That is a significant amount of sugar, particularly for a child, and especially upon waking in the morning.

The main point is that parents and guardians must take responsibility and not give children the opportunity to become accustomed to high-sugar breakfast cereals in the first place. In other words, do not regularly serve sweetened cereal to children for breakfast. If your child has already developed a preference for sugary cereal at breakfast, she can be re-trained. A preference for salty foods can be unlearned, even among adults; in the same way, the desire for sweetened breakfast cereal can be unhabituated. After regularly consuming unsweetened cereal for a while, her craving for a sweet sensation, particularly in the morning, will gradually diminish. Initially, a bowl of rather "plain" cereal topped with sliced bananas may not be bursting with flavor, but eventually, her taste buds will adjust and she will learn to like it. And in fact, she will probably notice that she feels better over time.

"Adult" Varieties of Breakfast Cereals

Please refer to Table 3, which compares the sugar and fiber content of several original cereals to their flavored/sweetened counterparts. Cereal manufacturers have started to target adults by introducing new flavors and sweetening up cereals that were originally wholesome "adult" versions. But due to one nutritional quality or another, these sweetened cereals often masquerade as "healthy" or "good for you," when they are actually high in sugar. As an example, flavors such as chocolate, caramel, and maple brown sugar are appearing more frequently amidst the once more nutritious brands. And companies are doing an incredible job of promoting these cereals to adults. Claims regarding weight loss, heart health, lower cholesterol, and digestive health abound on the front of cereal boxes and on advertisements. Obviously, these strategies are not aimed at youth. It is not that these claims are necessarily bad – in some cases this information aids in choosing the better or more appropriate option. As a warning, however, always be mindful. For instance, just because a cereal is a good source of fiber or antioxidants does not indicate that it is low in sugar. Likewise, a product that claims to aid in weight loss is not guaranteed to be high in fiber. A cereal packed with vitamins and minerals is not necessarily heart healthy. The list goes on and on. The key is to always read and compare nutrition facts labels and ingredients listings.

Food manufacturers commonly add items that sound nutritious, like yogurt, fruit, nuts, and/or "clusters" to sweeten up breakfast cereals. Yogurt, fruit, and nuts may be healthy in and of themselves, but when added to cereal, they are usually highly-processed and overly-sweetened, which contributes a significant amount of sugar to the cereal. In some cases, companies are simply making the cereals look and taste more appealing with items usually reserved for dessert, such as frosting, brown sugar, and flavorings like maple or vanilla. But because these are added to what is recognized as a nutritious cereal, it is oftentimes assumed that the more flavorful variety is still wholesome. On the contrary, when an original cereal is altered – such as by the addition of yogurt, fruit, clusters, and/or other types of flavorings – the sugar content of the cereal typically doubles, at the least (refer to Table 3).

TABLE 3: Comparison of Sugar and Fiber Content of Original Cereals and their Flavored/Sweetened Counterparts*

Cereal	Sugar per Serving (g)	Fiber per Serving (g)
Kellogg's' Special K'		
Original (per 1 cup serving)	4	0
Cinnamon Pecan (per ¾ cup serving)	7	3
Blueberry (per ¾ cup serving) Multigrain Oats & Honey (per 2/3 cup serving)	8	3
Red Berries (per 1 cup serving) Vanilla Almond (per ¾ cup serving) Chocolatey Delight (per ¾ cup serving)	9	3
Low-Fat Granola (per ½ cup serving)	9	5
Fruit & Yogurt (per ¾ cup serving)	10	3
General Mills Cheerios'		
Original (per 1 cup serving)	1	3
Duche de Leche (per ¾ cup serving)	6	2
Multi Grain (per 1 cup serving)	6	3
Oat Cluster Cheerios Crunch (per ¾ cup serving)	8	2
Frosted (per ¾ cup serving) Fruity (per ¾ cup serving) Banana Nut (per ¾ cup serving) Honey Nut (per ¾ cup serving) Yogurt Burst Strawberry (per ¾ cup serving) Chocolate (per ¾ cup serving) Multi Grain Peanut Butter (per ¾ cup serving)	9	2

Cinnamon Burst (per 1 cup serving)	9	5
Apple Cinnamon (per ¾ cup serving)	10	2
General Mills Chex˙		
Rice (per 1 cup serving)	2	1
Corn (per 1 cup serving)	3	2
Wheat (per ¾ cup serving)	5	6
Cinnamon (per ¾ cup serving) Chocolate (per ¾ cup serving)	8	1
Honey Nut (per ¾ cup serving)	9	1
Multi-Bran (per ¾ cup serving)	10	6
Post® Shredded Wheat˙		
Original (2 biscuits) Original Spoon Size (per 1 cup serving)	0	6
Shredded Wheat 'n Bran˙ (per 1¼ cup serving)	Less than 1	8
Lightly Frosted (per 1 cup serving) Honey Nut (per 1 cup serving)	12	6
General Mills Kix˙		
Original (per 1¼ cup serving)	3	3
Honey (per 1¼ cup serving)	6	3
Berry Berry (per 1¼ cup serving)	7	2
Kellogg's˙ Rice Krispies˙		
Original (per 1¼ cup serving)	4	Less than 1
Rice Krispies Treats˙ Cereal (per ¾ cup serving)	9	0
Frosted Krispies˙ (per ¾ cup serving)	12	0
Cocoa Krispies˙ (per ¾ cup serving)	12	Less than 1
Quaker˙ Life˙ Cereal		
Original (per ¾ cup serving)	6	2
Cinnamon (per ¾ cup serving) Maple & Brown Sugar (per ¾ cup serving)	8	2
Kellogg's˙ Mini-Wheats®		
Unfrosted Bite Size (30 biscuits)	0	8
Frosted Bite Size with Fruit in the Middle - Mixed Berry (24 biscuits)	10	6
Frosted Bite Size Original (about 21 biscuits) Frosted Little Bites® Original (42 biscuits)	11	6
Frosted Mini-Wheats® Big Bite Cereal (7 biscuits)	12	6

Frosted Mini-Wheats® Bite Size: • Strawberry Delight (about 25 biscuits) • Cinnamon Streusel (about 23 biscuits) • Blueberry Muffin (25 biscuits) • Maple & Brown Sugar (about 25 biscuits) Frosted Mini Wheats Little Bites® Cereal: • Chocolate (about 42 biscuits) • Cinnamon Roll (47 biscuits)	12	6
Post® Bran Flakes		
Original (per ¾ cup serving)	5	5
Raisin Bran (per 1 cup serving)	19	8
General Mills Fiber One˙		
Original (per ½ cup serving)	0	14
Honey Clusters (per 1 cup serving)	6	13
Caramel Delight (per 1 cup serving)	10	9
Frosted Shredded Wheat (per 1 cup serving)	12	9
Raisin Bran Clusters (per 1 cup serving)	14	11
General Mills Total˙		
Original Whole Grain (per ¾ cup serving)	5	3
Honey Almond Flax Plus+ (per 1 cup serving)	14	4
Raisin Bran (per 1 cup serving)	17	5
Kellogg's˙ Bran Cereals		
All-Bran® Complete® Wheat Flakes (per ¾ cup)	5	5
All-Bran® Original (per ½ cup serving)	6	10
All-Bran® Bran Buds® (per 1/3 cup serving)	8	13
Kellogg's Raisin Bran® Extra! (per 1 cup serving)	12	6
Kellogg's® Cracklin' Oat Bran® (per ¾ cup serv)	15	6
Kellogg's Raisin Bran® Cinnamon Almond (per 1¼ cup)	18	5
Kellogg's Raisin Bran˙ (per 1 cup serving)	18	7
Kellogg's Raisin Bran Crunch˙ (per 1 cup serving)	20	4

Cereal ingredients, formulations, and nutrition information may change. Please refer to current product packaging for the most accurate and up-to-date nutrition facts.

Hot Cereals

Table 4 provides a comparison between original and sweetened hot cereals in terms of sugar and fiber content. As can be deduced from the table, the most wholesome oatmeal is the original (plain and unsweetened) flavor. Both old-fashioned and quick oats in the canister cook within a few minutes in the microwave and contain purely one hundred percent whole grain oats with no sodium. Instant oatmeals in the packets, on the other hand, do contain additional ingredients, including salt. However, if you are desperate for convenience, original (unflavored, unsweetened) instant oatmeal is an acceptable option. With nine grams of sugar per serving, the Quaker® Apples and Cinnamon, Cinnamon and Spice, and Maple and Brown Sugar oatmeal flavors are acceptable occasionally, such as for a special breakfast on the weekend.

In regards to instant hot cereals, one packet is not satiating for many individuals, namely developing children and adolescents. Therefore, if your child requires more than one packet of instant oatmeal for breakfast, at least double the amount of sugar listed in Table 4 in order to determine the total quantity of sugar he would ingest.

The Weight Control® and lower-sugar oatmeals manufactured by Quaker® are good options for the adult segment of our population. The Weight Control® variety is an excellent source of fiber, very low in sugar, and provides protein; it is likely to fill you up and keep you satisfied through the morning. The lower-sugar oatmeals contain fifty percent less sugar than the regular full-sugar versions. The problem is that both of these types of oatmeal contain alternative sweeteners (such as acesulfame potassium and/or sucralose), making them inappropriate for children to consume on a regular basis, plus they remain highly sweet-tasting.

Another nutritious hot cereal is Cream of Wheat®; as with oatmeal, the healthiest options are the original unflavored varieties. The most wholesome Cream of Wheat® choices are the two-and-a-half minute original Whole Grain and instant original Healthy

Grain versions because they contain whole grains and are good sources of fiber. The two-and-a-half minute Cream of Wheat® cereals contain less salt than the instant kinds, yet still cook quickly in the microwave. Thus, the absolute best selection is two-and-a-half minute original Whole Grain Cream of Wheat®, because it contains significantly less sodium and a similar amount of fiber compared to the instant original Healthy Grain. However, if instant Cream of Wheat® is the only option for your family, with no sugar and six grams of fiber, instant original Healthy Grain is the top choice.

TABLE 4: Comparison of Sugar and Fiber Content of Hot Cereals and their Flavored/Sweetened Counterparts*

Oatmeal	Sugar (g)	Fiber (g)
Quaker' Instant Hot Oatmeal (Per Packet)		
Original	0	3
Maple & Brown Sugar Apples & Cinnamon Cinnamon & Spice	9	3
Raisin Date, & Walnut	11	3
Strawberries & Cream Peaches & Cream	12	2
Raisins & Spice	14	3
Quaker' Kids Mix-Up Creations™ Instant Hot Oatmeal (2 Pouches)		
Fruit Pancake	13	4
Quaker' True Delights Instant Hot Oatmeal (Per Packet)		
Wild Blueberry Muffin	9	4
Quaker' Heart Medley's™ Instant Hot Oatmeal (Per Packet)		
Apple Cranberry Almond	11	3
Banana Walnut	12	3
Cream of Wheat' Instant Hot Cereal (Per Packet)		
Original Healthy Grain	0	6
Original	0	1

Maple Brown Sugar Strawberries 'n Cream	13	1
Cinnamon Swirl Chocolate Cinnabon*	14	1
Apples 'n Cinnamon	16	1

Hot cereal ingredients, formulations, and nutrition information may change. Please refer to current product packaging for the most accurate and up-to-date nutrition facts.

Toaster Pastries and Strudels

It is utterly astounding that toaster pastries and toaster strudels® are marketed as breakfast items. The designation of "toaster" does not automatically transform a food into a beneficial part of the morning meal. Pastries and strudels, most of which are coated in frosting, are dessert items belonging in a bakery. Unfortunately, just as with sweetened cereals, these products are located on the lowest shelves of the breakfast aisles, in clear view and reach of children. Beyond being unacceptable for breakfast, these products are not even suitable as a snack. To prove this, simply review some of the flavors being displayed to kids on the bottom shelves; most sound like an ice cream flavor rather than a breakfast item: Frosted Chocolate, Chocolate Chip Cookie Dough, Cookies and Crème, Hot Fudge Sundae, Strawberry Milkshake, S'mores, and Boston Cream Pie.

Please refer to Table 5, which specifies the amounts of sugar, fiber, and fat present in selected toaster pastries. Although one brand does contain significantly less sugar than the others, it is higher in fat. Another brand offers a couple of low-fat options, but the sugar content remains high. Most are low in fiber; while a couple of varieties may be a good source of fiber, the high sugar content is not worth the trade-off. The bottom line is that toaster pastries and strudels are inappropriate as breakfast or snack items because they are high in sugar and/or fat, plus they taste really sweet. These products are only acceptable as a dessert.

TABLE 5: Comparison of Sugar, Fiber, and Fat Content of Selected Toaster Pastries*

Toaster Pastry	Sugar per Serving (g)	Fiber per Serving (g)	Fat per Serving (g)
Kellogg's® Pop-Tart® Toaster Pastries (Per Pastry)			
Frosted Strawberry Milkshake	11	1	5
Frosted Hot Fudge Sundae	12	2	5
Unfrosted Brown Sugar Cinnamon	12	Less than 1	8
Unfrosted Blueberry Unfrosted Strawberry	13	Less than 1	5
Frosted Cinnamon Roll	13	Less than 1	7
Frosted Apple Strudel	14	Less than 1	5
Low Fat Frosted Strawberry Low Fat Frosted Brown Sugar Cinnamon	15	3	2.5 and 3
Wildlicious® Frosted Wild! Grape Wildlicious® Frosted Wild! Strawberry Wildlicious® Frosted Wild! Fruit Fusion	15	Less than 1	5
Frosted Rainbow Cookie Sandwich˜	15	Less than 1	6
Frosted Brown Sugar Cinnamon	15	Less than 1	7
Frosted Strawberry Frosted Cherry Frosted Blueberry Frosted Raspberry	16	Less than 1	5
Frosted Chocolate Chip	17	Less than 1	6
Wildlicious® Frosted Wild! Berry Frosted Chocolate Chip Cookie Dough	18	Less than 1	5
Frosted S'mores	19	Less than 1	5
Frosted Cookies and Crème Frosted Chocolate Fudge	19	1	5
Pillsbury® Toaster Strudel® Pastries (Per Pastry)			
Boston Cream Pie	8	Less than 1	7
Cream Cheese and Strawberry	8	Less than 1	8
Danish Style Cream Cheese	8	Less than 1	9

Apple Blueberry Cherry Strawberry Raspberry Wildberry Apple Cream Danish	9	Less than 1	7
Cinnamon Roll with Brown Sugar	9	1	7
Nature's Path˚ Organic Toaster Pastries (Per Pastry)			
Frosted Cherry Pomegran™	17	1	4.5
Unfrosted Strawberry Unfrosted Blueberry Unfrosted Apple Cinnamon	18	1	4.5
Frosted Raspberry Frosted Chocolate Frosted Wildberry Acai	18	1	5
Frosted Strawberry	19	1	4
Frosted Blueberry	20	1	4
Frosted Brown Sugar Maple Cinnamon	20	1	4.5
Frosted Apple Cinnamon	21	1	4.5

* Toaster pastry ingredients, formulations, and nutrition information may change. Please refer to current product packaging for the most accurate and up-to-date nutrition facts.

Breakfast Bars and Snack Bars

For the most part, the breakfast bars, cereal bars, and various snack options manufactured by cereal companies are more appropriate for dessert than for breakfast or as a snack. While a sit-down, well-balanced meal or snack is always preferred to a pre-packaged item of any type, a healthy breakfast bar, granola bar, or medium-sized muffin is acceptable when absolutely necessary for an on-the-run breakfast or snack. However, finding a wholesome choice can be extremely difficult to do.

When selecting a breakfast bar, snack bar, or muffin, carefully read and compare the nutrition facts labels; the same guidelines for choosing a healthy breakfast cereal apply in this situation. Additionally, look for a product that does not contain any partially hydrogenated oils (a source of trans-fats). A single bar or muffin is rarely substantial on its own, especially when eaten for breakfast, and particularly for growing children and adolescents; pair one with nutritious items like fresh fruit and low-fat milk or yogurt.

There are a few bars and muffins on the market that do meet (or come very close to meeting) the nutritional criteria, however, they still taste overly sweet and are therefore unfitting for breakfast or as a snack. To clarify: any product drizzled, covered, or coated with some type of frosting or other sweet confection is too sweet to be consumed other than for dessert. Furthermore, any product that includes "chocolate," "mocha," "caramel," "cookies," or similar term as a descriptor is suitable solely as a treat. Also, read the ingredients listing and if sugar and/or other sweeteners, such as corn syrup or brown sugar, are listed in the first few ingredients and/or multiple times, that is a good indication that it better serves as a dessert item than as a breakfast or snack food. In addition, be wary of reduced-sugar products, as oftentimes these contain alternative sweeteners (such as sucralose), which are unsuitable for children.

Healthy Breakfast Ideas

A simple way to determine your family's breakfast habits is to ask, "Did my child eat breakfast this morning? If so, what did he or she have?" Next, question yourself, "Did I have breakfast this morning? If so, what did I eat?" As stated earlier, one of the most wholesome breakfast choices is unsweetened, low-fat, high-fiber cereal with low-fat (1%) or non-fat (skim) milk; add fresh fruit such as sliced banana, strawberries, or blueberries to flavor it naturally, as well as boost the nutritional value. Dried fruit, like raisins, and freeze-dried fruit are acceptable, but because they are high in (natural) sugar, use a small amount (one to one-and-a-half tablespoons) and alternate with fresh fruit mornings. For instance, if unable to give up your morning bowl of raisin bran, add up to one-and-half tablespoons of raisins to original (plain) bran flakes every other day. You will consume less sugar, and the homemade version is less processed than raisin bran that comes packaged in a box. On the alternate days, top original bran flakes or other fiber-rich cereal with fresh fruit. Similarly, original (unflavored) oatmeal and Cream of Wheat® can be topped with fresh fruit or a small amount of dried or freeze-dried fruit, along with some low-fat or non-fat milk. You may also occasionally sprinkle hot or cold cereal with up to one ounce of unsalted all-natural nuts, such as walnuts or almonds.

Next are some examples of breakfast cereals and various snack bars that meet the nutrition criteria, followed by additional breakfast ideas. Due to posing a potential risk of choking, some of the items listed are only appropriate for older children, adolescents, and adults; please always keep your child's age and stage of development in mind when selecting breakfast cereals and snacks.

Examples of breakfast cereals that meet nutritient recommendations:

- Original Cheerios®

- Wheat Chex®

- Corn Chex® or Rice Chex® mixed with a higher-fiber cereal, such as Wheat Chex®

- Original Shredded Wheat (spoon-/bite-sized is most appropriate for children and adolescents)

- Post® Shredded Wheat 'n Bran®

- Post® Grape-Nuts® or Grape-Nuts® Flakes

- Post® Original Bran Flakes

- Kellogg's® All-Bran® Original or Complete® Wheat Flakes

- Original Wheaties®

- Original Whole Grain Total®

- Quaker® Essentials™ Crunchy Corn Bran®

- Kashi® Original Go-Lean®

- Kashi® 7 Whole Grain Flakes or Nuggets

- Barbara's® Shredded Wheat or Shredded Spoonfuls Multigrain

- Barbara's® Original Puffins®

Examples of snack bars that meet nutritional recommendations:

- Kashi® TLC® Cereal Bars – with nine to ten grams of sugar, these are some of the lowest-sugar "cereal" bars on the market; these should be consumed occasionally only.

- Kashi® TLC® Chewy Granola Bars in the Peanut Butter, Honey Almond Flax, and Trail Mix flavors contain five grams of fat (zero saturated and trans fats), but they are relatively low in sugar and have a higher fiber and protein content compared to other granola bars, making them some of the most nutritionally acceptable granola bars available.

- Kashi® TLC® Pumpkin Pecan Layered Granola Bars have eight grams of sugar, but they are low in fat and a good source of fiber and protein, which makes them nutritionally superior to most other snack bars on the market.

- Among crunchy granola bars, Kashi® TLC® Honey Toasted 7 Grain Crunchy Granola Bars are a top choice. Although they contain eight grams of sugar and five grams of fat, this is less than similar bars, plus they are higher in fiber and protein than other crunchy varieties.

- Two-ounce VitaMuffins® or VitaTops® in non-dessert flavors, including BlueBran and CranBran. While some of these muffins contain a bit more than the ideal amount of sugar, they do not taste extremely sweet, are low in fat and high in fiber, and are packed with vitamins and minerals, so they are better options than many of the muffins on the market. (The sweeter varieties, like Deep Chocolate and Banana Choco Chip, are excellent choices for dessert.)

Further breakfast recommendations include one hundred percent whole grain (such as one hundred percent whole wheat) toast or bagels, and whole grain waffles that comply with the nutrition guidelines for cereal. For instance, Eggo® Nutri-Grain® Low-Fat Whole-Grain waffles; Van's™ Totally Natural Lite waffles made with whole grains; or Kashi® 7 Grain All Natural waffles. Suggested toppings are lower-salt natural peanut butter (with no more than fifty milligrams of sodium per serving) that contains no added sugar – although high in fat, it is healthy fat; apple butter; fruit spreads, such as Smucker's® Simply Fruit® Spreadable Fruit; reduced-sugar preserves (not sugar-free, which contain alternative sweeteners); or reduced-fat cream cheese. Because these condiments are concentrated sources of sugar and/or calories, the key is to use them sparingly rather than slather them on. In other words, pay close attention to serving sizes, which are generally one to two tablespoons, depending upon the product. If waffles are eaten at home, a couple of additional topping and dipping options are unsweetened natural applesauce and low-fat or non-fat vanilla or fruit-flavored yogurt. Again, use a modest amount, about one-fourth to one-half cup total (up to four ounces).

On a final note, it is not the case that higher-sugar or lower-fiber cereals, breakfast bars, granola bars, or muffins cannot ever be enjoyed. But they should not be eaten regularly. These options may be consumed occasionally, but should be reserved as a special treat, such as when on vacation or for dessert. Now that the importance of a well-balanced breakfast has been established, two more major components of children's and adolescent's diets are lunches and snacks. Just as a nutritious morning meal is essential, wholesome lunches and snacks are also imperative; the following chapter will explain how to make healthy lunches and snacks a reality for your family.

6 WHOLESOME LUNCHES & SNACKS

Eight year old James either buys lunch at school or takes something that is entirely pre-packaged, such as a Lunchable®. His mom and dad plainly tell him to make "healthy choices" at school, but he inevitably orders pizza, a cheeseburger, or chicken nuggets with French fries or tater tots. What does not help the situation is that James also takes a quick-grab convenience item for his morning snack at school: a bag of chips or cookies, a sweetened granola or cereal bar, fruit snacks, or a package of salty, high-fat crackers. Thankfully, he eats a well-rounded breakfast. But after lunchtime, James starts to feel irritable and fatigued. James and his parents do not realize that the foods he is eating for lunch and snack are highly processed; as a result, James consumes an excessive amount of sugar, fat, salt, and additives. Not only that, his intake of fiber, vitamins, and minerals is low. It is no wonder that James is moody and sluggish by the end of the day. Even though James eats a healthy breakfast and even a well-balanced dinner, his total intake of fruits, vegetables, and whole grains is inadequate because he ordinarily consumes unwholesome lunches and snacks.

The topic of lunches and snacks is complex, particularly because there are myriad options. Should children buy a lunch at school or bring a brown bag lunch from home? Which foods are most healthful in each instance? What is the long-term risk of choosing the most convenient options for a child's lunch?

The Third School Nutrition Dietary Assessment Study

In 2007, approximately sixty percent of all children and adolescents who attended a school participating in the National School Lunch Program purchased a school lunch on a given day.[1] While many school districts and schools are trying to implement healthier school lunch programs, unwholesome options abound. Foods that should not be consumed on a daily basis continue to be offered regularly, especially at the secondary level. Such items include pizza, hamburgers and cheeseburgers, chicken nuggets, hot dogs, corn dogs, and French fries – foods that children will routinely choose if given the option. In fact, even though most schools have nutritious lunch selections available, the majority of students continue to make unhealthy choices.[2] This is partly because it is difficult for schools to implement changes in ways that children will actually accept, and kids often opt for the less healthy items because they have not been taught otherwise. Regardless of the nutritional value, a large proportion of the items available in school cafeterias is highly processed and lacks freshness. For example, the third School Nutrition Dietary Assessment Study found that more than forty percent of school lunch entrées were commercially prepared rather than freshly prepared; these entrées were major sources of calories, total fat, saturated fat, and sodium.[3,4]

The third School Nutrition Dietary Assessment Study (SNDA-III) was conducted during the 2004-2005 school year; it represents all public schools participating in the National School Lunch Program and includes students in first through twelfth grades.[5] The purpose of the study was to examine the quality of meals provided by schools and whether or not they comply with nutrition standards.

Fat, Sodium, and Fiber Intake among Children and Adolescents

SNDA-III reveals that approximately eighty percent of all public school children and adolescents have a high intake of saturated fat while over ninety percent consume an excess amount of sodium.[6] Moreover, total fat, saturated fat, and sodium intakes tend to be highest among those who participate in the School Lunch Program. However, total fat intake is greatest among high schoolers, independent of whether or not they purchase a school lunch. Additionally, according to SNDA-IIII, about fifty percent of all children and adolescents do not consume an adequate amount of fiber, with fiber intake decreasing as children move from elementary school to middle school to high school; this includes both those who do and do not take part in the School Lunch Program.[7] Taken together, this evidence reveals an alarming trend: Youngsters are eating the type of diet that, over the long term, can lead to heart disease and a host of chronic ailments.

Sodium, Fiber, and Fat Content of School Lunches

School lunches typically contain very high levels of sodium, yet provide little fiber. Findings from SNDA-III show that virtually zero of the schools studied met sodium recommendations; in fact, the sodium content of lunches provided to students was nearly two times the recommended level.[8] In addition, few school lunches contain an adequate amount of fiber, largely because whole grain products are not widely available.[9] For instance, SNDA-III found that only five percent of the breads and rolls offered separately from an entrée contained any whole grains.[10] SNDA-III further reveals that the amount of total fat and saturated fat present in school lunches are usually higher than recommended.[11,12] Although most elementary and secondary schools do offer low-fat lunches or low-fat items, high-fat options are more prevalent and children usually choose the higher-fat foods.[13]

According to SNDA-III, the primary sources of total fat, saturated fat, and sodium in school lunches are: pizza; salad bars and entrée salads, such as a taco or chef's salad; Mexican foods, like tacos, burritos, and nachos; hamburgers, cheeseburgers, and other meat sandwiches; peanut butter sandwiches; French fries and similar potato products – baked or fried – especially in secondary schools; salad dressings; and condiments and spreads, such as mayonnaise, sour cream, or ranch dip.[14] Compounding the issue is that most of these items are not rich sources of fiber or other essential nutrients.

Fruit and Vegetable Consumption at School

SNDA-III confirms that the consumption of fruit and vegetables at school is low among all students and falls from an average of about a half-cup in elementary school to approximately one-third cup in high school.[15] Making matters worse is that, on average, around fifty percent of all children and adolescents do not eat any fruit, one hundred percent fruit juice, or vegetables (excluding French fries and similar potato products) at school. These numbers include children and adolescents who participate in the School Lunch Program and those who do not. Furthermore, one hundred percent fruit juice is consumed more frequently than whole fruit among middle school and high school students, with the majority of juice obtained at school rather than brought from home.[16]

While most schools provide some form of fruit, vegetable, or one hundred percent juice as part of a school lunch, SNDA-III reveals that more than forty percent did not offer fresh fruit or raw vegetables every day.[17] For example, canned fruit was served most often while fresh fruit was available for only half of all lunches.[18] Possibly even more concerning is that starchy vegetables, including French fries, corn, and potatoes/potato products, are the "vegetables" most often served and consumed at all school levels.[19] As discussed in chapter four, "Healthy Eating Habits Begin Early," French fries should never be considered a vegetable; beyond that, starchy corn and potatoes are inferior in nutritional value in comparison to deep-colored vegetables like spinach, broccoli, carrots, and tomatoes.

Competitive Foods

Competitive items are foods and beverages sold for lunch (or snack) at school, but that are not part of the National School Lunch Program. Examples of competitive foods include those sold à la carte in the school cafeteria, in vending machines, in school stores and snack bars, or for fundraisers. Unfortunately, competitive foods are widely available at all school levels. However, access to competitive foods becomes more prevalent as children move from elementary school to middle school to high school.

SNDA-III found that almost three-quarters of elementary schools, nearly all middle schools, and every single high school have at least one type of competitive food option.[20] More specifically, about two-thirds of elementary schools and nine out of ten middle and high schools have à la carte items available at lunch.[21,22] At the same time, vending machines are present in more than a quarter of elementary schools, over eighty-five percent of middle schools, and almost all high schools. These numbers are significant because it has been proven that greater access to competitive foods and beverages leads to an increased consumption of these items.[23] Analysis of SNDA-III demonstrates that forty percent of all students purchase at least one competitive product on a typical school day, with consumption lowest in elementary students and greatest among high schoolers.[24]

The widespread availability of competitive foods is a concern because the most commonly consumed competitive products are high-calorie, low-nutrient snack and dessert items, such as cookies, cakes, brownies, candy, and sports drinks.[25] These types of items are not only high in calories, sugar, and/or fat, but they promote the development of unhealthy eating habits among youth. Moreover, children and adolescents who eat competitive foods consume an average of at least one hundred and fifty calories from calorically-dense yet nutrient-poor items; if these empty calories are omitted from a child's diet, it could help prevent the development of overweight and obesity.[26] Besides, any item that can be stored in a vending machine, snack bar, or school store is highly processed, unwholesome, and lacks freshness, irrespective of its nutritional content.

A review of SNDA-III shows that only fifteen percent of all secondary schools with vending machines refrain from offering empty calorie foods and beverages in them.[27] SNDA-III also reveals that school vending machines do not usually provide water or one hundred percent juice any more frequently than other beverages, such as flavored milks, sports drinks, or carbonated beverages. Additionally, while lower-fat snack options are available in vending machines, they are not as common as the higher-fat versions. For instance, SNDA-III found that chips were available in thirty-four percent of high schools, but only six percent offered lower-fat varieties; twenty-three percent provided cake-type desserts, but only nine percent contained reduced-fat types.[28]

High-Calorie, Low-Nutrient Foods Consumed at School

According to SNDA-III, almost half of all children and adolescents in public school consume some type of high-calorie, low-nutrient food purchased at school on any given day.[29] The most frequent calorically-dense, nutrient-deficient foods obtained at school are baked sweets, like pastries, donuts, and cake-type desserts; dairy-based desserts such as ice cream; and French fries and similar potato products. The majority of these items are eaten at lunchtime. At all school levels, baked desserts and French fries/similar potato products provide over half of all the calories derived from high-calorie, nutrient-poor foods. Those who obtain and eat these types of foods at school consume an average of two-hundred calories from these items.[30] Just as with calories derived from competitive foods, eliminating these concentrated sources of calories from the diet would be sufficient to prevent overweight and obesity among children and adolescents. More than that, as consumption of foods packed with calories yet lacking in nutrients increases, vitamin and mineral intake decreases.[31,32]

Analysis of SNDA-III shows that children and adolescents who participate in the National School Lunch Program have a greater intake of baked goods and French fries (and similar potato products); at the secondary level, more dairy-based desserts, such as ice cream, are also consumed.[33] In fact, French fries and similar potato products are the top "vegetable" source of fiber.[34] SNDA-III reveals that snack items and desserts were available in close to forty percent of elementary school lunches, over forty percent of middle school lunches, and nearly half of high school lunches.[35] Brownies, cookies, and cakes are the most common desserts available. On a positive note, however, chips (other than tortilla chips) and juice drinks that are not one hundred percent juice are rarely included as part of a school lunch; when they are served, these items are more common at the secondary level than in elementary schools.

Association between Foods Sold at School and Body Weight

One SNDA-III study in particular demonstrates the relationship between elementary school lunches and body mass index (BMI). Even when controlling for multiple variables, children who attend elementary schools that serve French fries or similar potato products as part of a school lunch more than one time per week have a greater chance of being obese compared to those in schools where French fries are never offered or are only served once per week.[36] The same is true regarding desserts: students at elementary schools where desserts are served as part of a school lunch more than one time per week are more likely to be obese. This same investigation found that access to vending machines near the cafeteria and containing high-calorie, low-nutrient items results in higher BMIs among middle school students. This is similar to the finding that "junk food" in vending machines and school stores is associated with higher BMIs among adolescents.[37]

School Healthy Policies

The United States Government now requires that all school districts draft and abide by a Wellness Policy, which must include nutrition guidelines regarding competitive foods. However, the wording of these policies is often quite general while the weight that these policies carry varies widely across the country, from district to district, and school to school.[38] Some districts have worked diligently and made significant changes, but others have not.

Beverage companies have agreed to comply with strict regulations specifying what they will and will not sell in schools. In elementary and middle schools, beverage sizes are limited to eight and ten ounces, respectively, and the only beverages offered are bottled water, one hundred percent fruit juice, and low-fat or non-fat milk (regular and flavored). The serving size increases to twelve ounces in high schools where they also sell diet sodas, sports drinks, and low-calorie drinks containing less than ten calories per serving.

While this agreement is beneficial and certainly a step in the right direction, it is still somewhat lacking in that beverages containing unnecessary sugar (flavored milks and sports drinks) continue to be available in schools. However, the serving size limitations deserve recognition for reinforcing the critical importance of paying attention to portion sizes.

Unfortunately, merely banning or limiting the sale of certain sweetened beverages in schools will not make much more than a dent in the epidemic of childhood obesity. This truth is a validated by a risk analysis that was conducted using data from several credible studies. In examining the association between soft drinks sold in schools and adolescents' BMIs, researchers determined that regular sodas from school vending machines have little effect on adolescents' weight status.[39,40] Moreover, the findings show that removing regular sodas from the vending machines would have no effect on students' BMIs. The researchers concluded that it is unlikely that school policies restricting or banning the availability of soft drinks would dramatically influence the BMIs of adolescents. This may be at least partly related to the fact that, according to the assessment, carbonated sodas from vending machines account for only a small amount of adolescents' total soft drink intake. In fact, teenagers drink considerably more carbonated beverages at home than they do at school.

Sweetened Beverages Consumed Outside of School

Additional research confirms the fact that school policies alone are unlikely to have a noticeable impact on the childhood obesity crisis.

For example, an intervention to reduce obesity in Massachusetts middle schools demonstrates that, while school vending machines are associated with sweetened beverage consumption among youth, children's homes/families and fast-food restaurants may be larger suppliers of these drinks than schools.[41] Because of this, the study authors concluded that although school health policies are essential, their impact on the diets of children and adolescents may be minimal. Perhaps more importantly, parents and caregivers should assess all possible sources of sweetened beverages, such as the home and fast-food restaurants; further, policymakers need to consider limiting access to all types of sweetened beverages, including flavored milks and sports drinks.

According to SNDA-III, nearly seventy percent of children and adolescents drink a sweetened beverage during the day; half consume these sweet drinks at home compared to one quarter who drink them at school.[42] Similarly, some experts believe that while school wellness policies may aid in reducing children's intake of sweetened beverages at school, improvements must also made at home and locations such as fast-food restaurants, where sweet drinks and other calorie-dense but nutrient-poor foods are often consumed.[43] These researchers also stated that parental education and nutrition education are critical in helping children to establish healthy habits.

High-Calorie, Low-Nutrient Foods Consumed Outside of School

SNDA-III demonstrates that although children consume approximately one-third of their daily calories at school, the majority of their food is eaten at home.[44] More than that, the foods and beverages consumed at home are more likely to be high in calories and lacking in nutrients compared to items obtained at school. Researchers concluded that in order to reduce children's excessive intake of high-calorie yet low-nutrient foods, changes must be made at home.[45] This is because home is where the greatest number of total calories and calories from "junk foods," like sweetened beverages, chips, salty snacks, and baked treats, are consumed.

This is not to imply that school districts and schools should not implement health and wellness policies in order to combat childhood and adolescent obesity – they absolutely should. However, America cannot rely on schools to reverse the obesity epidemic because changes in schools alone will not solve the widespread problem. Changes definitely need to be made; anything and everything that might help teach and reinforce healthy habits to children and adolescents must be put into action, both at home, at school, and elsewhere. The concern is that society as a whole will be tempted to simply breathe a sigh of relief and think, "Okay, the schools are making changes, so we do not need to take further action or worry about obesity among our youth." On the contrary, it is imperative that changes begin at home.

Schools, communities, and homes (including parents, families, and caregivers) must forge a partnership. Children need to observe and learn healthy habits at home as well as at school. And it is critical that schools reinforce what is being taught at home. But of utmost importance is that parents, family members, and other primary caregivers set the foundation for a life of health and wellness among youth.

School Lunch Recommendations

Unless your child truly qualifies for a free or reduced-price school lunch, school lunches should be purchased occasionally only – at the most, approximately one time every week or two weeks. Eating foods purchased at school should be viewed like eating out: as an exception, a privilege, not the norm. Just as important, when you send your child to school with lunch money, ensure that he purchases a lunch that is part of the School Lunch Program rather than buying items à la carte or out of a vending machine, school store, or snack bar. Furthermore, discuss wholesome lunch options versus unhealthy choices and make sure he selects the most nutritious items available; if necessary, send a list of acceptable options from that day's lunch menu to school with your child. As an occasional treat, allow your child to pick one of his favorite foods, such as pizza or a hamburger, but no more than once every month or two months. And make sure he combines it with healthy accompaniments, like a nutritious side salad with low-fat/light dressing, fresh fruit, and low-fat plain (unflavored) milk or water. The main goal is to establish lifelong healthy eating habits in your child. Is he currently eating the type of lunch that will be beneficial for him to eat for the rest of his life? If not, consider making a few changes in order to provide him with more wholesome lunches.

Brown Bag Lunches

The concerns about lunch items available at school do not necessarily guarantee that a lunch sent from home is any healthier. Nowadays, lunches packed at home are often filled with quick, easy-to-grab convenience foods which are overly processed and, for the most part, unhealthy. In fact, in some cases a lunch served as part of the National School Lunch Program may actually be more nutritious than a lunch brought from home.[46] For instance, SNDA-III found that children who participate in the National School Lunch Program consume more fruits, vegetables, and milk – yet fewer desserts, snack items (including cookies, candy, and potato chips), and sweetened beverages – at lunchtime.[47] While those who do not eat a school lunch include students who purchase competitive foods, such as items à la carte and from a vending machine, or eat lunch off-campus, such as at a fast-food restaurant, this does include those who bring a brown bag lunch from home. SNDA-III also reveals that a large proportion of sweetened beverages (carbonated sodas, fruit drinks, lemonades, sweetened teas, and sports drinks) consumed at school are actually sent from home, particularly among elementary school students.[48]

Packing your child's lunches (or helping an older child pack her own lunch) gives you input about what she does – and does not – eat for lunch. It takes about five to ten minutes to prepare a nutritious lunch for your child when she is at home, so it makes sense to devote the same amount of time to packing her school lunch. Realistically, approximately ten minutes per lunch is not an enormous amount of time.

Although it takes little time, throwing an assortment of pre-packaged items into a lunch box does not qualify as packing a healthy lunch. Convenience foods and beverages are highly processed and usually full of calories, sugar, fat (especially saturated), and/or sodium, along with preservatives, additives, and other ingredients that are nearly impossible to pronounce; it is precisely these ingredients that transform a food into something that is quick to grab, easy to eat, and palatable. At the same time, these products tend to be low in vital nutrients, including fiber, vitamins, minerals, and disease-fighting antioxidants. On a regular basis, these products are toxic to anyone's body, particularly that of a developing child. Plus, an underlying goal is to help children develop an appreciation for the natural flavor of foods; this cannot be accomplished by serving convenience foods.

As you begin to send more healthful lunch and snack items, a key issue that needs to be addressed is the influence of peers. It is inevitable that your child will see other students purchasing pizza and French fries or bringing a Lunchable® and a sweetened beverage for lunch. Or eating a bag of cookies for snack. Be sure to sympathize and try to understand your child's perspective. As with all nutrition-related topics, an age-appropriate explanation as to why your child is served different lunch and snack foods can work wonders. Also, moderation is the key. As previously stated, allow your child to purchase pizza occasionally, or send a Lunchable® once in a very great while as a special treat. Discuss with your child why these items are to be eaten occasionally rather than every day, and why they are combined with wholesome options when they are consumed. Explain that a daily intake of processed foods rather than fresh, healthy choices like whole grains and fresh fruits and vegetables can result in low energy levels and illness, and over the long-term may lead to more serious conditions, like heart disease and cancer. Talk to your child about the rewards of eating healthy lunches and snacks: feeling great, having plenty of energy, demonstrating good behavior in the classroom, improved performance at school, and getting sick less often. There is even the possibility that after becoming accustomed to fresher wholesome foods and the knowledge of their benefits, your child will not enjoy the taste of processed foods as much.

Examples of Actual Lunches Sent to School

Studies are unnecessary to prove that many of the foods sent to school as part of a child's lunch are unwholesome and lack nutritional value. Simply walk through a school cafeteria or talk with teachers who observe what is sent from home on a daily basis. The following examples are actual lunches that have been packed at home and sent to school with a child.

- Three small slices of cheese pizza, leftover cold popcorn chicken and French fries, strawberry-flavored yogurt, and a cherry-lime-ade carbonated beverage

- A sandwich on white bread, a chocolate yogurt, a vanilla yogurt, and an orange-flavored Jell-O®. Note: the young child who brought this and the lunch above often packed her own lunches, but her mom or dad needed to either help her pack it or double-check to make sure what she packed was appropriate.

- A candy bar, some crackers, and a Dr. Pepper® soda

- A sandwich on white bread with a bag of chips on a daily basis

- Mini chocolate chip muffins, a package of fruit snacks, Jell-O®, and a Capri Sun®

- A plain jelly or Nutella® sandwich on white bread every day

- Mini pretzels, oyster crackers, and mini chocolate chip cookies

- Pre-packaged muffins, a squeezable yogurt, and a chocolate pudding daily

- A package of fruit snacks, a pudding, and a Twinkie®

- Cheetos®, a chocolate pudding, and a juice box

- A marshmallow creme sandwich, potato chips, fruit snacks, and chocolate milk

- A plain piece of white bread, Cheerios®, a package of chips, and popcorn; the reason being, "That is all he likes."

- Half of a sandwich, a Little Debbie® snack cake, six marshmallow Peeps®, and a Kool-Aid® juice box

A young boy in my daughter's preschool class had a pizza Lunchable® with apple juice for lunch every day. His mother reported, "That is all he will eat." This scenario is becoming increasingly common. As another example, the mother of a ten year old obese patient I worked with did not prepare healthy school lunches or snacks for him; as a result, he ate at least two packages of fruit snacks every day because his mom packed them in his lunches and served them as a snack. This type of eating pattern – regularly consuming quick, easy-to-grab convenience foods – was part of the reason this boy was obese and had other health issues at the age of ten.

A long-time teacher whose perspective I highly respect says, "I wonder where we are headed. I do not believe it when I hear a parent say, 'That is all my child will eat.' If parents do not enforce good nutrition at home, kids will not pick up good habits out in society. It has to start at home! I would love to see teachers follow through, but I do not see that happening either, so it is up to parents."

Healthy Brown Bag Lunches

Contrary to widespread belief, most children would eat healthier if they were simply given the opportunity. In many cases, a child's diet would improve dramatically if he was regularly offered fresh fruits and vegetables while at the same time served "junk food," like French fries, less frequently. For instance, SNDA-III demonstrated that fruit and vegetable consumption (excluding French fries and similar potato products) increased among elementary school students when fresh fruits and vegetables were available on a daily basis and French fries/similar potato products were not offered.[49] If your child is not currently accustomed to eating nutritious lunches, it may take time for him to accept the changes, but in many cases, he will grow to enjoy and appreciate the healthier, more wholesome foods you pack.

The first step in packing a healthy lunch is to involve your children; allow them to assist with planning and preparing their lunches in age-appropriate ways. With much parental guidance, especially initially, let your kids help decide what will go into their lunch boxes – both while shopping at the grocery store and at home making their lunches. This not only ensures that they will eat their lunches, but it teaches and reinforces positive eating habits. However, parents are the ultimate decision-makers regarding what is and is not appropriate to pack in a lunch, and oftentimes, children will eat what you send even if they complain about it at home. Also, allow children to pick out their lunch boxes at the beginning of the school year; this gives them ownership and increases the likelihood that they will eat what is in it. Use an insulated lunch bag with an ice pack to keep lunches cold as well as an insulated thermos when needed, such as for hot soup or a cold smoothie. As always, modify foods to your child's age and developmental abilities. Some of the following lunch recommendations may pose a choking hazard for young children.

A general rule of thumb for packing a well-balanced lunch is to include:

1. A "main dish," such as a sandwich or wrap, containing fiber-rich whole grains and a lean source of protein.

2. Fresh fruit or, occasionally, unsweetened natural applesauce or fruit canned in water, juice, or extra-light syrup.

3. At least one serving of fresh vegetables.

4. Another option is a serving of low-fat or non-fat dairy, such as yogurt, cottage cheese, or slices of reduced-fat natural cheese; if this makes your child's lunch too large, occasionally pack it in place of a fruit or vegetable and then be sure to send a fruit or vegetable as part of your child's snack.

5. A bottle of plain water.

Ingredients for a Healthy Lunch or Snack

- High-fiber whole grains (with two to three grams of fiber per slice, or three to five grams per serving, such as one hundred percent whole wheat): bread, bagels (try miniature bagels), tortillas, pita bread, and low-fat/baked, lower-sodium crackers, such as reduced-fat Triscuits® or whole grain rye crackers.

- Chopped or sliced fresh and skinless lean chicken or turkey breast.

- Lean, lower-sodium fresh and natural deli meat; while I recommend avoiding processed meats, if you buy packaged lunch meat, select brands that contain no more than twenty percent of the Daily Value for sodium (less than 480 milligrams) and are "natural," with minimal processing and preservatives.

- Low-sodium tuna fish (chunk light is lowest in mercury) or salmon canned in water; flaked fresh salmon or other fish.

- Natural nut butters: choose those that are lower in sodium, with no more than fifty milligrams of sodium per serving, and that contain no added sugar.

- Hummus or reduced-fat cream cheese, plain or flavored.

- Reduced-fat/light natural cheeses; avoid processed cheeses, like American.

- Low-fat or non-fat yogurt or cottage cheese, with or without fruit. Try serving plain, unflavored yogurt with fresh fruit, such as strawberries or blueberries; if your child is not accustomed to plain yogurt, it will take time for her taste buds to adjust, but she may very well learn to like it.

- A hard-boiled egg.

- Fresh fruit: bananas, apples, oranges, pears, grapes, peaches, nectarines, plums, kiwi, melon; be creative and try different varieties of your regular standbys or send something new, such as berries or cut-up mango or papaya.

- Fresh vegetables, plain or with a small amount of hummus or low-fat dip: baby carrots; carrot, celery, or jicama sticks; snap peas; sliced cucumber, mushrooms, or radish; chopped broccoli and/or cauliflower; bell pepper strips: red, yellow, orange, green; miniature tomatoes, such as cherry, grape, or plum.

- Pack dark-green lettuce or spinach/baby spinach leaves, tomato slices, and other vegetables in a separate container to be placed on top of a sandwich or wrap.

- Low-sodium vegetable juice or low-fat, reduced-sodium vegetable soup.

- A fun salad full of vegetables and other toppings your child enjoys.

- An occasional treat (no more than about once per week): two to three small cookies (Nilla* wafers, Ginger Snaps, and Animal "Crackers" are good choices because they are not overly sweet), a small homemade baked good, a few pieces of small candy, or a small serving (four to six ounces) of one hundred percent fruit juice.

- Other "treats" that may be sent more frequently include a special note from mom, dad, or other family members and stickers.

- Water is the best beverage choice; if your child does not consume an adequate amount of dairy (or calcium-rich dairy alternatives) each day, a serving of low-fat or non-fat plain milk may be an option (refer to chapter eight, "The Truth about Sweetened Beverages").

Healthy Lunch Box Ideas

- Homemade chicken salad (composed of lean skinless chicken breast, a small amount of low-fat or non-fat mayonnaise, and chopped celery) with spinach or dark green lettuce in a whole wheat pita; chopped watermelon; miniature tomatoes.

- Egg salad (made with one egg and a small amount of low-fat or non-fat mayonnaise and mustard) on whole grain bread; fresh red and green grapes; cucumber slices.

- A peanut butter and jelly (or peanut butter and honey, apple butter, or banana) sandwich made with lower-sodium natural peanut or other nut butter containing no added sugar on one hundred percent whole wheat bread slices, pita bread, or a tortilla; apple slices; raw broccoli with hummus.

- A lean turkey sandwich on a one hundred percent whole wheat bagel with dark green lettuce, tomato, a slice of reduced-fat/ light natural cheese, and a small amount of low-fat or non-fat mayonnaise or mustard; unsweetened natural applesauce; fresh snap peas.

- Low-fat, lower-sodium whole wheat or other whole grain crackers with: lean, lower-sodium natural deli meat and reduced-fat/light natural cheese OR reduced-fat cream cheese OR lower-sodium natural peanut or other nut butter (with no added sugar); orange slices; a simple tossed green salad with low-fat/light dressing.

- Tuna salad (prepared with low-sodium chunk light tuna canned in water and a small amount of low-fat or non-fat mayonnaise and chopped pickle; also try using salmon instead of tuna, flaked fresh or canned in water) with lettuce on whole grain bread; low-fat or non-fat cottage cheese; fruit canned in water, juice or extra-light syrup. Because lettuce is the only vegetable in this lunch, try to include a vegetable, such as baby carrots, with snack.

- Hummus on a whole grain pita or tortilla with baby spinach, tomato, cucumber, and/or other veggies as desired; chopped cantaloupe; slices of reduced-fat/light natural cheese.

- A whole wheat tortilla or pita stuffed with: lean, lower-sodium natural turkey, chicken, ham, or roast beef; reduced-fat cream cheese OR low-fat or non-fat mayonnaise or mustard and reduced-fat natural/light cheese; spinach, tomato, and/or other veggies such as avocado, olives, mushrooms, shredded carrot or cucumber, bell pepper strips, pepperoncini, or roasted red peppers. Make it simple: a whole wheat tortilla wrapped around meat, cheese, mustard, and spinach. Pair this wrap with some fresh fruit like strawberries.

- A whole wheat miniature bagel with reduced-fat cream cheese
OR low-fat or non-fat mayonnaise or mustard, lean and lower-
sodium natural deli meat OR hummus (no cream cheese,
mayonnaise, or mustard if using hummus), dark green lettuce or
baby spinach leaves, and other vegetables as desired. Pack low-
fat or non-fat yogurt and blueberries, too.

- A vegetable quesadilla (try using shredded or chopped carrots and
broccoli) with a light amount of reduced-fat cheese on a whole
grain tortilla. Kids love these and are unaware that they are eating
vegetables. Serve these quesadillas for dinner and then make and
send an extra one for lunch the next day. Include a serving of fruit,
such as chopped mango or papaya.

- A gourmet salad: start with a tossed dark-green leafy salad
with a variety of fresh vegetables. Then add items like chopped
lean meat; garbanzo, kidney, or other whole beans; baby corn
or corn kernels; shredded or diced reduced-fat/light natural
cheese; chunks of avocado or olives; or pieces of hard-boiled
egg. Consider topping it with some chopped fresh fruit, such
apples or pears, a sprinkling of dried fruit, like golden raisins
or Craisins*, or a pinch of chopped or slivered unsalted natural
nuts. Pack a small container of low-fat/light dressing separately,
along with some whole grain rye crackers and a plum.

- Whole wheat or other whole grain pasta with low-fat marinara
sauce, with or without chopped vegetables and/or lean ground
meat (in other words, leftover healthy spaghetti from dinner the
night before); low-fat or non-fat cottage cheese or yogurt; baby

carrots. When you send this type of lunch, ensure that the snack contains fruit.

- A slice of leftover vegetable pizza with light cheese on a thin or whole grain crust; a simple tossed green salad with low-fat/light dressing; low-sodium vegetable juice; kiwi slices.

- Low-fat, reduced-sodium vegetable chicken soup (packed in an insulated thermos); low-fat whole grain crackers with reduced-fat/light natural cheese; a pear.

- Low-fat, reduced-sodium lentil soup (in an insulated thermos); a freshly-baked low-fat, whole grain roll or slice of bread (occasionally bake homemade bread in the bread-maker); celery and/or carrot sticks with low-fat dip. Be sure to send fruit for snack time.

- Low-fat, reduced-sodium tomato soup (in an insulated thermos); lean natural deli meat with low-fat or non-fat mayonnaise or mustard and reduced-fat/light natural cheese on one hundred percent whole wheat bread; a peach or nectarine.

Snacks

SNDA-III confirms that snacking is very common among children and adolescents, and most often occurs at home.[50] SNDA-III results further show that the items that children and adolescents usually snack on tend to be high in calories, sugar, fat, and/or sodium and low in nutrients, whether they are obtained at home or at school. This is largely because the types of snack foods that are most often purchased by or for children and adolescents are convenience items: pre-packaged, highly processed, and unwholesome. As described previously, these products contain minimal nutritional value and may ultimately be hazardous to children's health.

Overall, the snacks that American youths typically consume require dramatic improvements. Just as with lunches, focus on the long-term goal: Do you want your child eating a pre-packaged bag of chips or cookies as a snack for the rest of his life? If not, it is time to re-think what he is eating at snack time, both at school and at home.

Examples of Actual Snacks sent to School

The teacher previously quoted reports that, although educators request for students to bring nutritious foods for snack time, more than half of the snacks that she encounters at school are unhealthy. According to her, "On the whole, the snacks that are sent to school are terrible!" The following are actual examples of snacks that children have brought to school from home; keep in mind that snack time often takes place during the morning hours.

- Brownies and similar baked desserts

- Sweetened dry cereals

- Pop Tarts®

- A bag of marshmallows

- Donuts

- Five Oreo® cookies

- Chocolate chip cookies and other types of cookies

- A package of fruit snacks

- Go-Gurt® (portable sweetened yogurt)

- Goldfish® crackers every day

- A bag of chips on a daily basis

Wholesome Snack Ideas

A nutritious snack generally contains fiber-rich whole grains, a moderate amount of lean protein, and fresh fruits or vegetables. Because snacks are often stored without an ice pack, it may be more difficult to include a protein source, which is okay. Many of the healthy lunch items carry over as wholesome snack foods, but there are a few additional suggestions.

- Whole grain brown rice cakes, unsalted or lightly salted

- Low-fat popcorn, air-popped or microwaved, preferably unsalted or lightly salted

- Dry cereal: low-fat, unsweetened, fiber-rich whole grain cereals such as Cheerios®, Quaker® Essentials™ Crunchy Corn Bran®, and Wheat, Corn, and Rice Chex®; refer to chapter five, "A Healthy Breakfast," for additional cereal recommendations

- Baked chips, occasionally

- A low-fat, unsweetened, high-fiber granola or cereal bar once in a while; see the previous chapter, "A Healthy Breakfast," for recommended snack bars

- Dried fruit: pay close attention to portion sizes because dried fruit is a concentrated source of sugar and calories

- Unsalted natural nuts and seeds, such as walnuts, almonds, pecans, or cashews. Serve a small amount (about one ounce) because although they are packed with nutrition, nuts are high in calories and (healthy) fat.

Examples of Healthy Snacks

- Half of a one hundred percent whole wheat bagel (regular or miniature-sized, depending upon child's age), with or without reduced-fat cream cheese, and fresh fruit, like grapes or berries, or fresh vegetables, such as baby carrots or miniature tomatoes.

- Baked chips with fresh salsa.

- Make your own wholesome trail mix with low-fat, unsweetened whole grain cereals (include at least one high-fiber brand, such as Cheerios® or Wheat Chex®), unsalted natural nuts, and dried fruit. Be creative and occasionally use types of cereal, nuts, or dried fruit that you do not normally use; in the case of nut allergies, this can also be made nut-free.

- Low-fat popcorn and a hard-boiled egg.

- Low-fat, lower-sodium whole grain crackers (such as reduced-fat Triscuits®) with slices of lean, lower-sodium natural deli meat and/or reduced-fat/light natural cheese.

- Spread celery and/or carrot sticks with reduced-fat plain cream cheese OR natural lower-sodium peanut or other nut butter containing no added sugar and top with raisins.

- Broccoli, carrots, and/or jicama with hummus or low-fat dip and low-fat whole grain crackers (or half of a whole grain bagel).

- Low-fat or non-fat cottage cheese or plain yogurt with fruit canned in water, juice, or extra-light syrup and a freshly-baked low-fat, whole grain muffin (occasionally make homemade muffins).

- A whole grain brown rice cake spread with natural lower-sodium, no-sugar-added peanut or other nut butter with apple or pear slices.

- A miniature orange, such as a tangerine, and a low-fat, unsweetened, high-fiber granola bar.

- Low-fat or non-fat (plain) yogurt topped with low-fat, unsweetened whole grain cereal along with a banana.

- A fruit smoothie: be creative and cater to individual preferences, but in general use low-fat or non-fat yogurt (vanilla or fruit-flavored), fresh or unsweetened frozen fruit, some ice cubes, and a splash of low-fat (1%) or non-fat (skim) milk. Pack this in an insulated thermos and send with an ice pack.

The good news is that, as the food industry attempts to manufacture a wider variety of convenience foods, more wholesome options without a plethora of additives are emerging. Examples include fresh sliced apples, baby carrots, or celery sticks in easy grab-and-go packaging; however, skip the dip that may accompany these products. Another choice is freeze-dried fruit, but these are concentrated sources of natural sugars, so serve these sparingly and occasionally only. Also, unsweetened natural applesauce is available in portable individual-serving containers. A word of caution: if you decide to purchase what appears to be a healthy convenience item regularly, check the ingredients listing to ensure that it does not contain any sugar, salt, fat, preservatives, or additives that are not present in the food's natural or original form.

Largely as a result of modern-day cultural influences, convenient lunches and snacks have become commonplace among children. Unfortunately, these quick and easy choices come at a high price, namely the health and well-being of children. To evaluate your child's lunch and snack habits, simply ask yourself, "What did my child eat for lunch today? What about as a snack? How many items came out of a bag or package that was torn open? How many times per week does he or she buy a lunch or snack at school, and what is usually purchased?" The bottom line is that regularly sending a child to school with money to buy a lunch or snack is not equivalent to providing a nutritious lunch or snack. But neither is packing easy, quick-to-grab products that are packed with additives and preservatives and may very well be less nutritious than many of the items for sale at school. Taking advantage of these convenient options once a month or every couple of weeks may be worthwhile, but not on a regular basis.

Although districts and schools are working to improve the nutritional value of the items they offer, many of the healthier items sold in school cafeterias or vending machines are not nearly as fresh and wholesome as foods that can be packed in a lunch sent from home. The key is to purchase and send fresh, nutritious items for your child's lunches and snacks, and to reserve the less-healthy, highly processed pre-packaged items for occasional use, when convenience is absolutely necessary or as a special treat for your child. Following lunch and snack times comes the dinner hour; this evening meal constitutes another predominant share of children's and adolescent's dietary intakes. As such, the next chapter will address the benefits gained from sitting down to healthy family meals coupled with eating out less frequently.

7 MORE FAMILY MEALS, LESS HAPPY MEALS®

Early Saturday morning, fourth grader José sits quietly in the back of his father's sedan as his family drives to his older brother's soccer game. On the way, they swing by the McDonald's® drive-through to grab a quick breakfast. After the game, they stop at Taco Bell® to pick up lunch as they head out to run errands. For dinner that evening, they order from Pizza Hut®. During the week, José's family is usually on-the-go, shuttling from one activity to the next; they frequent local fast-food drive-through windows an average of three, sometimes four, times per week. Family meals occur infrequently at his house, usually about once a week. Of predominant concern is that José believes this routine to be normal. In addition, he is starting to feel the effects of this type of diet: tired and lethargic as well as frequently experiencing illness, such as respiratory infections.

Not long ago, going out to eat was an infrequent luxury, whether it was at a sit-down or fast-food restaurant. Now the tables have turned, and for many families, eating out is the norm, while sitting down to a home-cooked meal has become a rare occasion. The issue is that routinely eating meals outside of the home negatively impacts the bodies and minds of children and adolescents. The excessive amounts of calories, fat, sodium, and sugar combined with the additives and preservatives present in these highly processed foods are harmful to health, particularly over time. More than that, when a child grows up accustomed to eating restaurant foods on a regular basis, he begins to believe that it is normal and acceptable to do so, a mindset that is insidiously toxic, especially as he approaches adolescence and adulthood.

The Increase in Eating Outside of the Home

Research proves that American families are eating meals obtained from outside of the home more often than in past decades. In 1970, one quarter of the total amount of money spent on food in our nation went towards eating outside of the home; less than thirty years later, this proportion nearly doubled and almost half of the entire sum spent on food was for eating out.[1] In as little as two decades, the percent of total calories that Americans obtained from restaurant and fast-food sources practically tripled, jumping from eight to twenty-two percent.[2] And there are no signs that this trend is going to slow. Thirty percent of Americans reported that eating at a restaurant or fast-food establishment is *necessary* for their lifestyle, and sixty percent indicated that they would frequent fast-food restaurants about as often as they did the previous year.[3]

More specifically, the frequency with which Americans visit fast-food establishments is on the rise; concomitantly, fast-food restaurants have proliferated. In 1970, there were approximately thirty thousand fast-food establishments in this country; in 1980, that number had jumped to about one hundred and forty thousand; as of 2001, there were around 222 thousand fast-food restaurants in the United States.[4] Additionally, at the end of the 1970s, only three percent of Americans' total daily calories came from fast-food; in just under twenty years, that percentage quadrupled with fast-food accounting for twelve percent of our daily calorie intake.[5]

Children and Adolescents

Unfortunately, children and adolescents are not exempt from our culture's new-found reliance on eating out, and their bodies and health are suffering. According to The Bogalusa Heart Study, the proportion of children consuming a meal at a restaurant jumped from a scant 0.3 percent to nearly five-and-a-half percent over the course of two decades.[6] In particular, the number of children eating dinner outside of the home more than tripled, increasing from about five-and-a-half percent to almost twenty percent during that same time period. Moreover, in the late 1970s, children consumed seventeen percent of their meals outside of the home; about twenty years later, the percentage of meals children ate away from home had practically doubled, reaching thirty percent.[7]

Over the course of twenty years, the sheer quantity of food consumed by children at restaurants increased an astonishing ten-fold, from 0.4 percent of the total amount of food they consumed in a day to four percent.[8] Predictably, the number of calories children and adolescents obtain from foods consumed at restaurants has risen over the years while the amount of calories derived from foods eaten at home has decreased. For example, at the end of the 1970s, fast-food comprised only two percent of the total calories ingested by children and adolescents; by the end of the 1990s, fast-food accounted for ten percent of their total calorie intake.[9] That is a five-fold increase in only two decades.

Eating out appears to occur more commonly among older children and adolescents. One survey found that approximately seventy-five percent of eleven to eighteen year olds ate at a fast-food restaurant in the previous week.[10] On average, adolescents frequent fast-food locales two times a week.[11] This is partly due to the fact that many well-known fast-food chains employ clever marketing techniques. It is believed that their selection of sites for new franchise opportunities is not arbitrary. Quite the opposite has been found: these restaurants may actually target locations near schools, even within walking distance.[12]

The Health Effects of Eating Out

Never mind the impact on a family's pocketbook, there are definite health consequences, both short- and long-term, to frequently ingesting meals obtained outside of the home. Eating restaurant foods, particularly fast-food, has been shown to result in a higher intake of calories, total fat, saturated fat, cholesterol, sodium, and sugar; a decreased consumption of fiber, calcium, and iron; and a lower intake of critical antioxidants, including beta-carotene and vitamins A and C.[13,14] Part of the problem is that restaurants generally serve large portions of high-calorie, low-nutrient foods. Research has found that visiting a fast-food restaurant usually leads to a greater consumption of French fries, carbonated soda and other sweetened beverages, cheeseburgers, and pizza; consequently, it typically results in a lower intake of fruit, vegetables, and milk.[15] If consumed on a regular basis, this type of diet places an individual at risk of not only obesity, but for developing a chronic health condition, such as heart disease, cancer, or osteoporosis.

Depending upon the particular restaurant and specific items ordered, a large fast-food meal (excluding dessert) might have as many as fifteen hundred calories and fifty-five grams of total fat while providing very little fiber or other essential nutrients. Put another way, this single fast-food meal virtually meets the calorie and fat needs of many average Americans for an entire day, yet contains very little nutritional value. In addition, the meal could contain at least half of an individual's daily sodium requirements.

To be more precise, a small serving of French fries by itself contains over two-hundred calories and ten grams of fat, and a large burger may have close to six-hundred calories and thirty grams of fat. Combine these two items, and your child is going to choke down eight-hundred calories and forty grams of fat before even adding a condiment like ketchup or a thirst-quenching beverage to the equation. These two foods alone provide close to fifty percent of a typical American's daily calorie requirements, and well over half of her daily fat needs. It is no wonder that heart disease and other nutrition-related ailments are on the rise.

Compounding the problem is that restaurants are a quickly growing source of sweetened beverages, supplying nearly one-quarter of all carbonated drinks consumed by children and adolescents.[16]

These are the main beverages served by restaurants, so eating out – especially fast-food – leads to a greater consumption of sweetened drinks. Research proves that the number of times a child or adolescent eats at a fast-food restaurant is directly related to the amount of sweetened beverages he consumes.[17] Stated another way, a child who eats at a fast-food restaurant one time per week is likely to ingest more sweet drinks than a child who does not eat at a fast-food restaurant at all; a child who visits a fast-food establishment twice a week will probably drink a greater amount of sweetened beverages than a child who eats there once per week, and so on. The negative effects of drinking excessive amounts of sweet beverages are discussed in the following chapter, "The Truth about Sweetened Beverages."

Eating Out and Obesity

According to experts, an over-consumption of fast-food and sweetened sodas is a contributing factor to the epidemic of obesity currently plaguing our nation.[18] Research demonstrates that there is a relationship between fast-food consumption and an individual's total calorie intake and weight status. For example, one study found that girls who eat fast-food four times per week ingest approximately 185 to 260 more calories per day than those who do not.[19] Over a short period of time, these extra calories can add up to excess body weight. Furthermore, studies show that meals and snacks consumed outside of the home are higher in calories than those eaten at home.[20] It is logical to conclude that if children and adolescents normally ingest high-calorie, high-fat restaurant foods, they are at a higher risk of becoming overweight.

Recommendations for Eating Out

There are a number of ways to make more nutritious choices when eating out, which will be discussed shortly. More important, however, is to limit the frequency with which your family eats out, and to increase the number of meals that your family shares together at home. This is because even the best choices at the healthiest restaurants have more calories and fat – and cost more – than a home-cooked meal.

For numerous health reasons, it is wise to limit the number of times your child eats outside of the home to one to two times each week, at most. Traditional fast-food establishments, including pizza parlors, should be visited no more than once every two weeks (twice a month). However, if weight is or could become an issue with any member of the family, I generally recommend eating out only one time per week or less, with fast-food kept to a maximum of once a month. If your child orders lunch at school during the week at all, this should be taken into consideration when making decisions regarding eating out.

In those instances when "fast-food" is actually a necessity, opt for contemporary take-out locales that offer healthy options, such as sandwich bars, taco bars, and Asian restaurants. The key, though, is to make the best possible selections because meals at these restaurants can be just as unhealthy as those at traditional fast-food restaurants. Examples include requesting little or no cheese, mustard instead of mayonnaise, whole beans versus refried, grilled or baked all-white skinless chicken breast, lean turkey breast, extra vegetables, brown rice, baked chips, and so on. Skip the high-calorie but low-nutrient items, such as sweetened beverages and desserts, altogether.

When eating at a sit-down restaurant, visit those that have the most nutritious choices available, and then exercise those healthy options the majority of the time. Special occasions should be celebrated, which often includes eating foods that are not usually consumed but are truly enjoyed; a favorite food or dessert, for instance. By all means, treat yourself and your family once in a while. Eating healthfully is about balance, moderation, and variety, as well as heeding internal hunger and fullness cues, even when eating out.

Of course, if your child or any family member is overweight, or at-risk of being so, these recommendations are rather general; each situation varies and recommendations need to be individualized to the person and family. In these cases, please seek the help of a registered dietitian with expertise in this area.

Eating Out Healthfully

The primary goal is to limit your family's consumption of restaurant foods, fast-food and otherwise. But when you do eat out, there are several ways to do so more healthfully. First of all, allow children of all ages to order a half-portion, or share a meal, from the adult menu rather than ordering off of the kids' menu. Children's menus usually consist of greasy unwholesome foods, such as chicken nuggets, a grilled cheese sandwich, or a cheeseburger and French fries. However, there are many additional ways to make your family's dining-out experience as healthy as possible.

- Become aware of where calories and fat are found in restaurant foods; be assertive and ask how foods are prepared and request ingredients and preparation methods that limit excess calories and fat.

- Look for terms indicating that a food is prepared with little or no fat. Examples include: baked, boiled, grilled, braised, roasted, poached, steamed, blackened, broiled without butter, charbroiled, stir fried, marinated in vinegar, and marinara or red sauce.

- Be wary of descriptions that indicate a food has been prepared with significant amounts of fat. Examples are: fried, deep fried, battered, breaded, buttered, buttery, pastry, golden brown, sautéed, marinated in oil, basted (with fat), scalloped, au gratin, gravy, Hollandaise sauce, Béarnaise sauce, Alfredo sauce, cheese sauce, rich, creamy, creamed, cream sauce, and á la mode.

- Patronize restaurants that offer heart healthy, low-fat, or light menu selections; choose from among these options.

- Avoid all-you-can eat buffets and unlimited salad bars – these quickly add up to excess calories.

- Plan ahead. Do not leave the house or enter a restaurant feeling starved; you are more likely to eat the first foods in sight as well as overeat due to being famished. If your restaurant meal will be higher in calories and fat, try to eat lighter, healthier foods during the rest of the day.

- Start with a lighter item, such as a tossed green salad with low-fat/light dressing or a broth soup. This will help provide satiety and prevent you from overeating higher-calorie foods.

- Eat judiciously – or not at all – from the bread or chip basket; avoid or limit butter and high-calorie, high-fat spreads and toppings.

- Whenever possible, order a healthy appetizer as a meal, a half-portion, a child-sized serving of a healthy meal, or share the meal.

- Do not become a member of the "clean plate club." Take leftovers home for lunch or dinner the following day.

- Drink plenty of plain water before and during the meal. Avoid alcohol and sweetened beverages.

- Pace yourself: try to be the slowest eater at the table. Put down your fork, converse, sip water.

- Order salad dressing, sauces, butter, sour cream, guacamole, cheese, and other condiments on the side and then use them sparingly, if at all.

- Ask that cheese, "special sauces," and mayonnaise be left off of sandwiches and burgers; request low-fat or non-fat mayonnaise, mustard, ketchup, pickles, and other low-calorie condiments instead.

- Choose vegetables that are prepared with herbs, spices, or olive oil; avoid those that are cooked with butter, cheese, or sour cream.

- Instead of French fries, try low-fat yogurt, fresh fruit, a green salad with low-fat/light dressing on the side, or a plain baked potato with salsa or another healthy topping.

- Avoid foods with a mayonnaise base, like potato or macaroni salad, chicken or tuna salad, and coleslaw.

- Whenever possible, opt for whole grains, such as one hundred percent whole wheat or rye bread, whole wheat pasta, brown rice, and oatmeal.

- Choose lean meats. Remove any skin from chicken or turkey and trim all visible fat from meats.

- Rather than ordering a cheeseburger or sandwich with "the works," select a small plain hamburger or turkey sandwich and pile on the vegetables.

- Order a pizza topped with vegetables and request extra vegetables. Opt for Canadian bacon rather than high-fat meats like pepperoni or sausage. Ask for half of the amount or a "light" amount of cheese. Choose thin and/or whole grain crust. Rather than ordering pizza from a restaurant, however, turn it into a family event and make your own healthier version at home.

- Only order dessert if you truly have room for it. Share your dessert or satisfy your sweet tooth with low-fat frozen yogurt, sorbet, or fruit.

- For breakfast, choose an unsweetened, low-fat, high-fiber whole grain cereal (hot or cold) with low-fat or non-fat milk; dry whole wheat toast, bagel, or English muffin with fruit preserves; fresh fruit; and/or low-fat yogurt. Avoid eggs, sausage, bacon, breakfast sandwiches, donuts, muffins, and pastries.

- Refer to the nutrition information that is available on most restaurants' websites or at the restaurant.

The Decrease in Family Meals

It is impossible to deny the fact that family meals are occurring less frequently in America. Lack of time is a primary reason that families do not prepare and sit down to healthy dinners anymore. Even when there is time, parents and guardians are often too tired because of other commitments like work, meetings, and children's sports and activities. Because there has been a surge in the availability of convenience foods, including fast-food and meals out of a box, can, freezer, or microwave, families have come to rely on these unwholesome options instead. As a matter of fact, research has found that whether or not a family sits down together for a meal is directly related to the mother's employment status. Family meals occur most often in homes where the mom is not employed, and are least common in homes where Mom works full-time.[21]

Family meals have become less and less common over the last few decades, corresponding with the growing rates of overweight and obesity in our nation. A national survey of over one thousand American women reveals that, when they were growing up, ninety-one percent of women routinely took part in family dinners; once they had their own families, though, only eighty percent of these women normally sat down for dinner with their families.[22] Furthermore, the percentage of women who reported eating family dinners was notably higher among the women in their sixties and seventies than those in their twenties and thirties.

The Bogalusa Heart Study found that over the course of twenty years, the proportion of children eating dinner at home fell from nearly ninety percent to approximately seventy-six percent.[23] In fact, according to telephone interviews conducted on behalf of several leading health organizations, including the National Center for Nutrition and Dietetics and the President's Council on Health and Fitness, the number of nine to fifteen year olds eating dinner with their families decreased by five percent in as little as four years.[24] Researchers blame changes in American society for the diminishing occurrence of family meals: a growing number of after-school activities, alterations in the structure and living arrangements of families, a greater availability of convenience foods, and the increased frequency of eating meals away from home.[25]

Family Dinners and Adolescents

For obvious reasons, the most common meal that families share with one another is dinner. But such family dinners tend to occur less frequently as children get older, with the most severe decline occurring in adolescence. Surveys have found that while, on average, nearly forty-five percent of families with young children eat a daily family dinner, only twenty-seven percent of families with twelve to seventeen year olds do so.[26] Parents spend more time eating with their younger children than their teenagers largely because family members tend to become busier and have conflicting schedules as children get older; this is probably related to growing independence among adolescents.[27]

The Growing Up Today Study, composed of more than sixteen thousand nine to fourteen year old children, demonstrates an age-related decline in the frequency of family dinner consumption, with the drop most prevalent in older children.[28] According to the results, over half of nine year olds eat a family dinner every day compared to only about one-third of fourteen year olds. A gradual decrease in the frequency of family meals has also been found in adolescents between the ages of twelve and seventeen: Compared to twelve year olds, about half as many seventeen year olds eat a nightly dinner with their families during a typical week (fifty percent versus twenty-seven percent, respectively).[29]

Similarly, the older the teenager, the less likely he is to sit down for a family meal. Project EAT (Eating Among Teens) reveals that middle school students take part in family meals much more frequently than high schoolers do.[30] Likewise, Project EAT demonstrates that young adolescents participate in family meals more often than those who are older: Almost sixty percent of seventh through ninth graders report eating five or more meals with their family per week in comparison to less than forty percent of those in tenth through twelfth grades.[31]

As youths move through childhood and adolescence, the nutritional quality of their diets becomes poorer, especially in regards to fruit and vegetable intake.[32] For example, according to the Centers for Disease Control and Prevention, nine out of ten high school students do not eat enough fruits and vegetables.[33] A lack of family meals contributes to the inadequacy of older children's and adolescent's diets, demonstrating the necessity for families to eat together more often.[34] This issue is similar to the problem with breakfast-skipping among adolescents; because the dietary patterns of adolescents are likely to carry over into their adult lives, it is imperative to focus on nutrition issues – such as sitting down for family meals – during this crucial period, if not beforehand.

On a positive note, there are several reassuring facts. First of all, a majority of parents and adolescents believe that family dinners are important, and family meals have not become obsolete.[35,36] In fact, as many as seventy-four percent of adolescents report that they enjoy eating dinner with their families.[37] Although it varies based upon age and gender, studies show that approximately one-third to one-half of children and adolescents regularly participate in family meals.[38,39] However, far too many youths still report few to no family meals each week: about one-third, according to research.[40,41]

Family Meals and Health

Routinely sharing meals as a family results in improved health on multiple levels. Families who regularly eat together tend to have healthier diets, and studies reveal that family meals have a remarkable impact on the nutritional quality of children's and adolescent's diets. Further, families that eat together at least five times per week are twenty-five percent less likely to encounter any type of nutritional health issue than those who do so once or less per week.[42]

Improved Dietary Quality

Normally sitting down for family meals increases the probability that children and adolescents will make wise food choices.[43] For instance, a majority of seventh and tenth grade students report that they would eat healthier if they ate with their families more often.[44] Additionally, research shows that family meals are the number one influence that parents have on how well adolescents eat.[45]

Studies demonstrate that family meals are associated with an increased intake of fruits, vegetables, calcium-rich foods, and grains as well as a decreased consumption of fried foods and soda.[46,47] Findings also reveal a higher intake of essential nutrients, including protein, fiber, calcium, folate, iron, and vitamins A, B_6, B_{12}, C, and E, among those who frequently sit down to family dinners. More than that, the diets of children and adolescents who regularly partake in meals with their families tend to be lower in saturated and trans fats, as well as provide a lesser glycemic load.[48] Glycemic load is the measure of a food's ability to raise an individual's blood sugar level. It encompasses both the quality and quantity of carbohydrate ingested and the body's resultant requirement for insulin. The bottom line: A high glycemic load may be related to an increased risk of developing type 2 diabetes.

Sitting down to family meals also helps establish and reinforce regular eating habits among children and adolescents. As an example, frequent consumption of family dinners results in a reduced intake of ready-made dinners such as frozen meals, SpaghettiOs®, and microwaveable entrees.[49] Another study found that adolescents who eat at least seven family meals per week consume less snack foods than those who engage in fewer family meals.[50] In addition, children and adolescents who share family meals at least three times per week are almost twenty-five percent more likely to eat nutritious foods, including fruits and vegetables, and twenty percent less likely to eat unwholesome foods, such as fast-food, soda, fried food, and candy/sweets, than those who take part in family meals less often.[51]

It is reasonable to conclude from this information that children and adolescents, as well as adults, who regularly sit down to family dinners are less likely to become overweight or obese. Studies confirm it.

Prevention of Obesity

Sitting down to a meal and conversing and interacting with family members, while not distracted by the television or other technology, causes children to eat more slowly and pay closer attention to their internal feelings of hunger and fullness; this usually results in the ingestion of more nutritious foods and decreases the likelihood of overeating. As introduced in chapter four, "Healthy Eating Habits Begin Early," the critical habit of sensing and responding to the body's hunger and fullness signals needs to be encouraged and reinforced during every stage of life.

According to research, four year olds who eat dinner with their families at least five nights per week are twenty-three percent less likely to be obese.[52] This correlation remains just as strong after accounting for other factors, such as socioeconomic status and maternal obesity, and was true even among preschoolers who were at high risk for obesity. Further, the Early Childhood Longitudinal Study (Kindergarten Cohort), which followed eight thousand children from kindergarten through third grade, demonstrates that children who consume the fewest family meals and watch the most television are at the greatest risk of obesity.[53]

The Growing Up Today Study, conducted among nine to fourteen year olds, found that children and adolescents who routinely sit down to family dinners have the lowest body mass indexes (BMIs), while those that eat family dinners infrequently have higher BMIs.[54] Additional research reveals that the more often children between nine and fourteen years of age take part in family dinners, the less likely they are to be overweight or obese.[55] In fact, enjoying family meals "every day" or "most days" reduces the risk of being overweight by fifteen percent compared to those who eat them "never or some days"; this is regardless of other possible contributing factors, such as physical activity level, total calorie intake, and time spent watching television or playing video games. Overall, studies show that children and adolescents who participate in at least three family meals per week are twelve percent less likely to be overweight than those who eat family meals less often.[56]

As if research does not provide sufficient evidence regarding the importance of regularly sitting down to family meals, the reality of not doing so speaks for itself. One of my saddest cases was an obese fifth grader whose single mother was unaware of the importance of preparing healthy meals for her family. Thus, they did not sit down together to eat and usually consumed meals in front of the television. This child's dietary intake was extremely poor: his diet predominantly consisted of highly processed foods, such as Chef Boyardee®, SpaghettiOs®, and hot dogs; he had a very low intake of vegetables and fiber; and he consumed excessive amounts of fat. As a result, this child became severely obese with elevated cholesterol and triglyceride levels, putting him at high risk for developing heart disease.

Protection against Unhealthy Dietary Habits

Regularly taking part in family meals protects children and adolescents from developing unhealthy eating habits and eating disorders. An inverse relationship has been established between frequent family meals and unhealthy dietary habits, such as skipping breakfast.[57] Engaging in family meals has also been associated with a lower occurrence of unsafe weight control practices.[58] Moreover, adolescents who normally eat family meals, place a high priority on family meals, and experience a positive, structured meal environment are less likely to suffer from disordered eating, even after controlling for familial factors, such as family unity.[59] One study shows that routinely participating family meals "while growing up" correlates with a lower risk of bulimia in adolescence; this association remains true even after taking additional factors into account, including family conflict and connectedness.[60] A review of the research demonstrates that adolescents who share family meals at least five times per week are thirty-five percent less likely to suffer from disordered eating, including bingeing and purging, self-induced vomiting, fasting, ingestion of diet pills, use of laxatives, and meal skipping.[61]

Additional Benefits of Family Meals

The benefits of regularly sitting down to family meals extend far beyond improvements in nutritional intake and physical health. Family meals build connectedness and unity between family members, promote psychological and emotional well-being, enhance academic performance, and provide an opportunity for parents to teach and serve as role models for their children.

Familial Interaction and Bonding

According to researchers, over half of all adolescents – including both those in early and late adolescence – think of mealtimes as a time to talk with other family members.[62] Hence, family meals are ideal for facilitating interaction and communication amongst family members, as well as fostering a sense of belonging and togetherness. Eating together aids in the development of a family's social relationship and promotes feelings of community and family identity. The unity and bonding experienced during family meals is especially critical during adolescence but also provides the structure and connectedness younger children need to feel secure.

Family meals offer order, routine, and consistency, something many children and adolescents sorely lack as modern-day American life grows increasingly busy and stressful.[63] Mothering mentors Elisa Morgan and Carol Kuykendall state in their book, *What Every Child Needs*, that, "One of the simplest ways to maintain a sense of family unity and belonging is to sit around a table together for a meal."[64] They expand, "Since plenty of distractions eat away at this family tradition, you need to be intentional – often sacrifice other things – to make it work. So turn off the TV. Set the table with candles. Make conversation the focus of the meal. Keep the communication positive. Involve each family member. Take turns cooking. Hold hands and say grace together, alternating who prays each time. Enlist children in preparation and cleanup."

Eating meals together as a family is a simple but effective strategy for maintaining communication and involvement with your children, especially as they reach adolescence and begin to establish their independence. Family meals enable parents and guardians to get to know their kids better and develop closer relationships with them. Compared to adolescents who eat less than three family dinners each week, those that participate in five to seven family dinners a week are more likely to talk to their parents about what is going on in their lives.[65] Parents who rarely take part in dinner with their families often report that they have a fair or poor relationship with their teenager; do not know or do not know well the parents of their adolescent's friends; and do not know the names of their teenager's teachers.[66] Moreover, adolescents who regularly eat family dinners typically state that they have excellent relationships with their parents, while teenagers who have infrequent family dinners are significantly more likely to report fair or poor relationships with their parents.[67]

Psychological and Emotional Health

Research shows that family meals contribute positively to the psychological and emotional development of young people, and it appears that consistently engaging in family meals helps them become better adjusted. For example, family connectedness, which is strengthened by sharing meals together, has been associated with healthy development among youth.[68] This includes a decreased risk of emotional problems, drug use, violent behaviors, unsafe methods of weight control, sexual activity, and suicidal tendencies. Further, regularly participating in family meals results in a lower incidence of depression and suicidal thoughts among both males and females, as well as a decreased likelihood of low self-esteem and suicide attempts among females.

According to surveys conducted by the National Center on Addiction and Substance Abuse at Columbia University (CASA),

children and teenagers who habitually eat dinner with their families
have a considerably lower probability of engaging in risky behaviors:
they are significantly less likely to smoke cigarettes, drink alcohol, or
use drugs.[69] Possibly more compelling is the finding that teenagers
who rarely or never eat dinner with their parents are more than
twice as likely to report that they plan on trying drugs in the future.[70]
These facts alone confirm the obligation to regularly enjoy meals
together as a family.

Improved School Performance

Research demonstrates that routinely participating in family meals
results in an improved performance at school. For instance, youths
who consistently sit down to meals with their families spend greater
amounts of time completing homework and reading for pleasure.[71]
Moreover, adolescents that partake in regular family meals are more
likely to earn better grades and have a higher grade point average.
Taking part in family meals has even been found to enhance a
child's language and literacy skills.[72] Additionally, CASA reports
that teenagers who have infrequent family dinners are more likely to
receive lower grades in school: Adolescents that eat less than three
family dinners per week are almost two times more likely to report
that they receive Cs and below than those who eat five to seven
family dinners each week.[73]

A Teaching Opportunity

Family meals provide an invaluable opportunity for parents to teach
and role model desirable behaviors to their children, including
manners, communication skills, nutrition, and healthy eating

habits.[74] In fact, participating in family meals can encourage children and adolescents to become interested in and knowledgeable about nutrition and health. For example, a couple of studies found that the regular occurrence of family dinners among school-aged children correlates with greater amounts of conversation and knowledge about nutrition-related topics.[75] The research also shows that over seventy-five percent of nine to fifteen year olds acknowledge their parents to be a source of information regarding nutrition, and ninety-eight percent found the information obtained from their parents to be valuable. Parents and guardians must take advantage of these truths and talk to their children and adolescents about nutrition and health, particularly while around the dinner table consuming a healthy meal, as well as while in the kitchen during meal preparation.

Making Family Meals a Priority

Based upon the research, sharing at least four to five family meals per week appears to confer the greatest benefits; I highly recommend aiming towards five a week. If not for the prevention of obesity, then for the countless other benefits that these meals offer to each family member. However, if your family currently consumes zero to two family meals per week, it is more realistic to gradually work up to three to four family meals per week, at least initially.

Considering the multitude of benefits to be realized when family meals are enjoyed frequently, it is well worth the extra time and effort to ensure that your family sits down to as many meals as possible each week. For this to happen, family meals must become a priority: Families must make time to sit down and eat together on a routine basis. In one study, both adolescents and parents reported that more frequent family meals were resultant of making them a higher priority, as well as not watching television during mealtime.[76]

A chief constraint for many families is that they are constantly on-the-go and lack the time necessary for family meals. The first step in resolving this issue is to recognize the obstacles to family meals in your household. Why is your family unable to sit down to family meals on a nightly basis? Once the barriers are identified, you can work to overcome them – either by removing them completely or working around them.

This will be discussed in more detail in chapter eleven, "Healthy Sleep, Rest, and Relaxation Habits," but in many cases, families are simply too busy with overloaded schedules. In these instances, families need to slow down instead of continuously running from one activity, event, or meeting to the next. As a result, family members will be home for meals on a more regular basis. However, there will invariably be times when schedules interfere with family mealtimes, and in these cases, families need to plan ahead, think creatively, and be flexible.

Plan Ahead

In order for meals to become a habit, families must be both purposeful and strategic; family meals will not happen based on good intentions alone. Prior to planning your meals for the next week and making your weekly shopping trip, evaluate your calendar. How many nights – and which ones – are extraordinarily busy? What do you want to do on those nights? On the other nights, is there anything special or new you would like to prepare? What are some of your family's favorite meals? What do you need to buy in order to make these meals? Your meal plan for the next week does not have to be written out and you are not bound to it, but having a general idea about what you are going to do will be exceedingly helpful.

In general, shop for groceries only once per week. Make a master grocery list of all the items you usually buy and print it out; to save time in the future, print out multiple copies, one for each upcoming week. As much as possible, organize this list according to your grocery store's layout in order to simplify the shopping trip. Be sure to save the list so you can make changes and print it out as needed. Also, ensure there are some blank lines in each category. Now you can quickly and easily mark the items you need to purchase each week, as well as add items that you may not ordinarily buy.

As often as possible, complete part of your meal preparation ahead of time, when there is time to spare and you are not rushed to get a meal on the table. For example, most vegetables can be chopped in advance and then stored in tightly sealed containers in the refrigerator; meat can be pre-cooked and then frozen or refrigerated, depending upon when it will be used; cheese can be shredded or sliced in advance, then stored in the freezer long-term or the refrigerator short-term.

Develop a repertoire of at least five quick and easy healthy meals that can be prepared in thirty minutes or less; keep the ingredients on-hand in the pantry and freezer. For example, stock the pantry with whole wheat spaghetti noodles and jars of marinara sauce, and have extra-lean ground turkey breast available in the freezer; add to that green leaf lettuce and tomatoes from the refrigerator. A spaghetti dinner with green salad awaits. Another idea is to keep whole wheat tortillas stored in the fridge. These can be filled with practically anything and become a well-rounded meal. Take, for instance, whole black beans or non-fat refried beans, instant brown rice, skinless all-white chicken breast, reduced-fat natural cheese, hummus, or avocado; top this with a variety of vegetables, such as baby spinach, chopped tomatoes, and red pepper spears. Combine the wrap with some fresh fruit and low-fat cottage cheese and you have a convenient wholesome meal. These become your "go-to" meals for those nights that are busier than usual.

It is acceptable to keep a couple of packaged or frozen meals on-hand that can be thrown together at a moment's notice, but these should be used only when absolutely necessary, no more than one time per week. Additionally, look for the most wholesome and nutritious options, such as those that are low in fat and sodium, high in fiber, minimally processed, and contain the fewest additives and preservatives, including being free of monosodium glutamate (MSG). It is worthwhile to pay a little bit more in order to purchase a higher-quality product; it will still be less expensive than eating out. Chop and toss in some extra vegetables or serve it with a green salad to create a more healthy and substantial meal.

Prepare a double recipe one to two times a week, or on the weekend, when you have some extra time. Freeze the extra meal so that you can pull it out whenever you lack the time to put an entire meal together. As previously mentioned, another option is to cook and freeze extra portions of a meal, such as the ground meat when you are making spaghetti; next week, just pull the cooked meat out of the freezer and put it in the refrigerator to thaw for taco night.

Think Creatively

One way to make meal planning simple is to create a weekly theme night. For instance, Monday night is Italian/pasta night, Tuesday is taco (or other Mexican fare) night, Fridays are homemade pizza night, Saturdays are burgers, steaks, or kebabs on the grill, and so on. In many cases, you can make the dinner more fun and interactive – and easier to prepare – by involving the entire family, such as by letting the kids fill their own tacos or build their own pizzas with a variety of healthy toppings.

For nights when you do not feel like cooking or are on-the-go, plan a couple of easy, quick dinners: Sunday evenings could be "gourmet" grilled cheese sandwiches with a hearty, wholesome vegetable soup, Wednesdays might be whole grain tortillas wrapped around reduced-fat natural cheese, lean meat, and fresh vegetables alongside baked potato chips or baked tortilla chips and salsa. Bear in mind, these nights are not set in stone and are interchangeable. For example, if your daughter has an unexpected soccer game on your regularly scheduled taco night, swap tacos with something that can be prepared more quickly, such as grilled cheese sandwiches and soup.

Include one or two monthly theme nights, such as serving a healthy breakfast for dinner. Regularly give each family member a turn to plan his or her favorite menu and involve the whole family in the preparation. Also, plan times to try new ethnic cuisines, such as Indian, Latin, or Greek.

Serving a fresh green salad and/or other vegetables with dinner is an ideal habit. However, there are bound to be nights when there is simply not enough time to prepare a salad or vegetable dish. In these cases, think outside of the box and serve a more convenient alternative instead, such as raw vegetables with low-fat/light dip.

Be Flexible

As often as possible, schedule your family's activities around your normal family dinner time, not vice versa. For example, if an activity or class you want to take occurs during your dinner hour, find another class time or choose not to participate. Unfortunately, this is not always realistic, especially as kids get older and become involved in organized sports and other activities. Decreasing your family's number of commitments will make this easier. As you work to make family meals the priority, this dilemma will become less common, and you can better navigate your way through it.

Keep in mind, though, that there is more than one way to cook a wholesome meal. Most families own a crockpot, but rarely use it. What is more, there is a plethora of cookbooks dedicated solely to cooking in a crockpot. This combination makes preparing an entire healthy meal simple and fast. A multiple tiered food steamer is another worthwhile investment. You can simultaneously cook fish or other lean meat, rice, and fresh vegetables with the touch of a button and then go help your kids with homework or clean the house. In addition, use your grill as often as possible, especially during the spring and summer months. Grilling on the barbecue can be a quick, easy way to create nutritious meals. A bread machine is also a straightforward and stress-free – yet invaluable – tool for baking fresh, wholesome, delicious breads. Be adaptable and innovative; think beyond your "status quo."

In order to accommodate your family's schedule, there are going to be times when everyone will need to be flexible. For instance, there may be evenings when you need to change the time that your family typically eats dinner so that every family member can be present, such as by moving it up an hour and making it an early dinner. Or plan a "family lunch" on Sunday afternoon when everyone is guaranteed to be home. Another alternative is to pack a healthy meal to take with you, and then eat it together between your children's activities; however, the requirement is that you sit down together as a family while you eat, not while driving in the car.

Remember, a family meal does not always have to be dinner. A family breakfast or lunch on a Saturday, or an early family dinner on a Sunday afternoon are excellent ways to connect with one other and can be wonderful occasions to eat healthfully while modeling appropriate eating habits and social skills.

Additional Recommendations for Family Meals

Turn Off All Distractions

Family meals must be technology-free. This means completely turning off all televisions, radios, computers, video games, phones, cellular phones, and texting devices. These electronic distractions detract from the sense of togetherness, quash mealtime conversation altogether, and lead to a decreased awareness of biological hunger and fullness cues. Always sit down around the table for family meals, and ensure that all technological devices are not only turned off, but that they are out of eyesight and earshot.

Involve the Entire Family

There is a desperate need for parents to teach children to cook – to plan and prepare balanced meals – and to do so healthfully. Kids need to grow up with the knowledge and ability to create nutritious meals so that one day they can do so for themselves and their own families. Moreover, one study found that adolescents who frequently participate in meal preparation make more healthful food choices.[77] However, today's culture no longer recognizes the importance of this vital skill.

There are numerous age-appropriate ways to involve children and adolescents in the preparation of family meals, and doing so enhances family bonding and feelings of togetherness. Thus, it is important to encourage all family members to participate in meal planning, shopping, and preparation; also, include everyone in the brainstorming of ways to make your family's meals more healthful.

Make It an Enjoyable, Positive Experience

The goal of family meals must be pleasure and enjoyment.[78] It is imperative that parents and guardians require positive interactions during family mealtimes. Conversations should be uplifting and encouraging. A good rule of thumb is to focus on the good things that happened during the day, as well as the activities that family members are looking forward to. Appropriate questions to ask are, "What are you thankful for today?" or "What was the best part of your day?" Avoid conflicts and arguments over sensitive topics such as grades, discipline, or money. Discussing controversial topics or expressing criticism only causes tension and makes the meal an unpleasant experience for everyone.

Set a Good Example

Children and adolescents are more likely to make family meals a priority if they see their parents doing the same. Parents can have an enormous impact on kids by planning, preparing, encouraging, and serving healthy meals that include a variety of nutritious foods. When parents actually sit down and eat these meals with their children, the benefits increase exponentially.

Perhaps the most stunning case I have encountered was an obese single father who was only thirty-three years old. He was diagnosed with a fatty liver due exclusively to an unhealthy diet. This man did not sit down to eat his lunch, which was typically composed of fast-food or easy-to-grab convenience foods, but instead ate while he worked. For dinner, he usually picked up fast-food on his way home from work, but if not, he haphazardly ate convenience foods throughout the night, such as frozen meals and Top Ramen®, rather than preparing a well-rounded evening meal. Alarmingly, his two year old daughter was already overweight as a result of her father's lifestyle. Remarkably, this man lost almost fifteen pounds over the course of one month by improving his diet, including a decreased consumption of fast-food and convenience foods, and by adding very modest amounts of exercise to his weekly routine.

While thankfully this father made enormous strides for his and his daughter's benefit, it is entirely possible to prevent this type of scenario in the first place. Start by asking yourself a couple of questions: "How many of my child's meals were obtained at a fast-food restaurant this week? What about from any type of restaurant?" Then transition to family meals: "How many times did my family sit down together for a meal this week? And how many of those meals were composed of items that did not originate from a can, box, freezer, or microwave?" From there, you can begin to initiate changes that will benefit your entire family in a number of ways. So now that the facts about eating out and family meals have been addressed, the next chapter will uncover the truth about sweetened beverages and discuss their contribution to the obesity epidemic.

8 THE TRUTH ABOUT SWEETENED BEVERAGES

Jacqueline, who is five years old, rarely drinks plain water. In fact, when her mother stops to think about it, Jacqueline virtually never consumes water. For breakfast, she is served one hundred percent apple or orange juice; her parents believe they are doing a good thing by providing her with a serving of fruit. For her morning snack, she usually has juice again. At lunchtime, she drinks a Capri Sun® or other type of fruit-flavored beverage. For her afternoon snack, she typically grabs a juice box. With dinner, she has milk – sometimes plain, but usually chocolate or strawberry flavored. When Jacqueline gets thirsty between meals and snacks, she gets herself a can of soda, a Capri Sun®, or a juice box. Her parents do not realize that over the course of a day, her sugar intake from sweetened beverages adds up significantly. More than that, Jacqueline often lacks an appetite for food because she has filled up on sugary liquids. Her weight is starting to sneak above what is healthy for her, and her parents are at a loss because, as they state, "She eats hardly anything!"

Oftentimes, the drinks that are served to children as an accompaniment to their meals and snacks are sweetened beverages, typically in some type of portable container. This is especially true when children eat pre-packaged convenience foods or meals from a restaurant, further making it an unwholesome meal or snack. The term "sweetened beverage" can convey a variety of meanings. To clarify, in this chapter, "sweetened beverages" refers to regular (non-diet) carbonated beverages, fruit-flavored drinks, fruit punch, lemonade, sports drinks, and flavored milks (such as chocolate or strawberry), as well as tea or coffee (iced and hot) with added sugar. The term does not include one hundred percent fruit juice, which was mentioned in chapter four, "Healthy Eating Habits Begin Early," and will be further discussed later in this chapter. Plain white milk is also excluded and will be addressed towards the end of this chapter as well.

Increased Consumption of Sweetened Beverages

Americans today, including children and adolescents, drink considerably more sweetened beverages and less plain milk than in past decades. For instance, research shows that the intake of sweetened beverages among Americans increased by one hundred and thirty-five percent between 1977 and 2001.[1] Conversely, milk intake fell by thirty-eight percent over the same time period. Most significant was a heightened consumption of carbonated sodas followed by fruit-flavored drinks. Furthermore, the average daily caloric intake in the United States has increased by 150 to 300 calories in the last twenty to thirty years; approximately half of these additional calories are derived from sweetened beverages.[2] The United States Department of Agriculture (USDA) reports that, per person, the consumption of carbonated drinks increased by nearly five hundred percent over the course of fifty years.[3] More than that, about half of all Americans drink beverages such as carbonated sodas or fruit drinks on a daily basis, and the majority are sweetened rather than diet. As will be discussed in detail, considerable evidence demonstrates that the intake of sweetened beverages has risen dramatically even among children and adolescents in recent decades. This shift towards a greater consumption of sweetened beverages correlates with the surge in rates of overweight and obesity in our country.

Toddlers and Young Children

The Feeding Infants and Toddler Study (FITS), introduced in chapter four, found that forty percent of toddlers between fifteen and twenty-four months of age consume fruit drinks other than one hundred percent fruit juice and more than eleven percent drink carbonated beverages.[4] The numbers do not improve as children get older: a National Health and Nutrition Examination Survey (NHANES) found that forty-four percent of young children between the ages of two and five consume fruit-flavored beverages other than one hundred percent fruit juice and thirty-nine percent drink carbonated sodas.[5] Of further concern is that these children consume fruit drinks in greater amounts than they do one hundred percent fruit juice.

As noted in chapter four, the dietary patterns and food preferences that toddlers and young children develop are likely to remain throughout childhood, and probably even beyond. Thus, the beverage habits and preferences that children establish before the age of two are critical, not only for the child's immediate health, but also to ensure the development of healthy dietary habits that are likely persist through childhood and adolescence.

Children and Adolescents

National surveys reveal that the number of six to seventeen year olds who drink carbonated beverages (including flavored waters and juice drinks that are carbonated) rose by almost fifty percent over two decades.[6] The percent of calories obtained from carbonated drinks among youths doubled during this time – from about three percent to approximately six percent per person. According to the findings, children's homes are the largest source of carbonated drinks; restaurants (fast-food and otherwise) are also major suppliers. Survey data also confirm that diet and sugar-free versions account for a very small proportion of kids' total beverage intake.

Research shows that in a thirty year time span, daily sweetened beverage consumption among eleven to eighteen year old adolescents rose dramatically: it doubled among girls and increased by more than two-and-a-half times among boys.[7] Similar to findings from other studies, milk intake decreased during the same period.

According to a Policy Statement issued by the American Academy of Pediatrics (AAP), fifty-six to eight-five percent of school-aged children and adolescents drink at least one carbonated beverage per day, and most are regular/non-diet.[8] Adolescent males tend to consume the greatest amounts, with one out of every five drinking four or more servings per day. Moreover, it has been reported that the majority of adolescents – sixty-five percent of

girls and seventy-four percent of boys – drink beverages such
as carbonated sodas or fruit drinks every day, most of which are
sweetened as opposed to sugar-free.[9]

There are several theories for the dramatic rise in sweetened
beverage consumption among youth in recent years: increased
marketing and advertising geared towards kids, widespread
availability, affordability, the ever-growing size of individual
containers, and more frequent visits to fast-food and other
restaurants where carbonated soda is a popular choice.[10]

Consumption of Greater Quantities

Americans are drinking greater volumes of sweetened beverages than
ever before. For example, between the late 1970s and the end of the
1990s, daily carbonated beverage consumption climbed from five to
twelve ounces, more than doubling.[11] Among youths who regularly
ingest these beverages, the amount consumed in the late nineties
(twenty-one ounces) was significantly greater than at the end of the
seventies (fourteen ounces). Research also demonstrates that from
1991 to 1995, consumption of carbonated drinks increased from
approximately six-and-a-half ounces to slightly over nine ounces
among the general population, and from about eleven-and-a-half
ounces to a little over nineteen ounces among adolescent boys.[12]

The Bogalusa Heart Study, which examined the meal patterns
of ten year old children over a twenty-year time period, found that
although the number of children drinking sweetened beverages
decreased, the total amount consumed rose dramatically.[13] This
reveals that children are drinking larger quantities of sweetened

beverages than in the past. The investigation also determined that milk consumption fell – there was a decline in both the percentage of ten year olds who drank milk as well as the amount of milk consumed.

A major factor contributing to the consumption of greater amounts of sweetened beverages is that larger volumes are now being packaged into individual containers. Individual-sized containers have grown exponentially over past decades: from six-and-a-half ounces in the 1950s up to twelve ounces in the 1960s, then to twenty ounces by the end of the 1990s.[14] Nowadays, there is the option of as many as twenty-four ounces. And what happened to six-packs of twelve-ounce cans? It seems that today's standards are twelve-, twenty-four-, and thirty-six packs.

Adverse Health Effects

Sweetened beverages are an exceptionally insidious poison because they are easily ingested and taste really good, but contain minimal – if any – nutritional value. Over a prolonged amount of time, an excessive amount of sugar is harmful to every cell in the body, leading not only to obesity and tooth decay, but causing increased triglyceride levels, metabolic abnormalities, and decreased nutrient intakes.[15] A steady intake of sweetened beverages delivers a daily dose of this deleterious sugar to children's bodies. Studies prove that there is an association between sweetened beverage consumption and adverse nutrition and health outcomes, including a greater intake of sugar and calories, overweight and obesity, lower nutrient intakes, poor bone and oral health, and an increased risk of diabetes.

Increased Sugar and Calorie Intake

Between 1977 and 1996, the ingestion of sweeteners such as sugar and high-fructose corn syrup rose by eighty-three calories per person, per day.[16] The vast majority (almost eighty-one percent) of these extra calories are due to an increased consumption of sweetened beverages. Sweetened drinks, especially regular/non-diet carbonated sodas, are the top contributors of added sugars to the American diet.[17,18] In fact, sweetened beverages are the primary source of added sugars in children's diets.[19] These large amounts of sugars supplied by sweetened beverages, such as carbonated sodas or fruit-flavored drinks, can result in an excessive calorie intake and quickly lead to preventable weight gain.

According to research, carbonated sodas contribute approximately thirty-six and fifty-eight grams of added sugar per day to the diets of adolescent girls and boys, respectively; depending on an individual's daily caloric needs, this nears or exceeds the USDA's recommendations for total added sugar intake per day.[20] Furthermore, between 1999 and 2004, American youth consumed an average of nearly two hundred and twenty-five calories from sweetened beverages each day.[21]

Individuals who regularly drink non-diet sodas have a greater daily calorie intake than those who do not.[22] For example, one study demonstrates that total calorie intake is approximately ten percent higher in school-aged children who routinely consume carbonated drinks compared to those who do not.[23,24] The National Heart, Lung, and Blood Institute (NHLBI) Growth and Health

Study, which followed over two thousand females from childhood to adolescence, shows that as sweetened beverage consumption increases, so does total calorie intake.[25] NHANES researchers discovered that a greater consumption of beverages – whether carbonated soda, fruit drinks, one hundred percent fruit juice, or milk – correlates with a higher intake of calories among preschoolers between two and five years of age.[26]

Overweight and Obesity

Several experts theorize that the increased consumption of sweetened beverages seen in recent years, especially carbonated sodas, may partly explain the growing rates of overweight and obesity among youth.[27,28] A higher intake of sweetened beverages is definitely a contributing factor to the multifaceted epidemic this country is facing. It is certainly not the only reason, because there is no single cause – and in some cases it may not even be a primary influence. But in nutrition counseling, an excessive consumption of sweet drinks is commonly encountered among overweight patients of all ages.

Consider this: a twelve-ounce can of soda, which is a small amount compared to the larger individual-sized containers widely available today, contains approximately one hundred and fifty calories and the equivalent of about ten teaspoons of sugar.[29] Added to the normal diet, one can of soda each day would result in a weight gain of fifteen pounds over the course of one year, or about one pound every three-and-a-half weeks.

According to research, there is a relationship between the consumption of sweetened beverages and weight gain, a higher body mass index (BMI), and overweight/obesity among children and adolescents. For instance, compared to children of a healthy weight, overweight children and adolescents are more likely to drink sweetened beverages.[30] Similarly, data obtained from NHANES reveal that overweight children and adolescents tend to consume more calories from drinks, particularly carbonated sodas, than those who are not overweight.[31] In addition, the Growing Up Today Study found that girls between nine and fourteen years of age who drink large quantities of sweetened beverages have higher BMIs and body weights than those who drink less or none at all.[32]

Results from a study consisting of more than ten thousand preschoolers suggest that sweet drinks, including one hundred percent fruit juice, are associated with weight status, especially among youngsters who are already obese or at high risk of obesity. Compared to those drinking less than one sweetened beverage per day, two and three year olds who were obese or at-risk of obesity at the beginning of the year-long study were about twice as likely to be obese at the end of the study if they consumed one or more sweetened beverages per day.[33]

Several long-term studies show that when children or adolescents increase their intake of sweetened drinks, over time, they experience greater weight gain, larger increases in BMI, and a higher risk of overweight or obesity than those who do not.[34] In addition, the Bogalusa Heart Study reveals that beverages containing added sugar (carbonated sodas, fruit-flavored drinks, tea, or coffee) are associated with the incidence of overweight among children.[35]

An experimental study conducted among school-aged children (seven to eleven year olds) proves that school-based programs designed to reduce children's intake of sweetened drinks can be successful. Over the course of one school year, an educational program resulted in the reduction of children's carbonated beverage consumption, which corresponded with a decrease in the number of overweight and obese children.[36] Furthermore, research has confirmed that there is a beneficial effect on body weights and BMIs when adolescents who frequently drink sweetened beverages reduce their consumption, especially among those with higher body weights and BMIs to begin with.[37]

Perhaps most convincing are results from the Planet Health intervention and evaluation project in which middle school students' risk of obesity increased sixty percent for each additional serving of sweetened drink consumed per day over the course of two school years.[38] This association remained significant after other possible causes were taken into account. Along with increased risk of obesity, researchers observed greater calorie intakes and higher BMIs among those who drank more sweetened beverages. The study authors concluded that consumption of sweetened drinks could be a contributing factor to the epidemic of childhood obesity.

Mentioned earlier, findings of the NHLBI Growth and Health Study aptly summarize many of the points in this section and reiterates a few main ideas suggested by this book. It was a ten-year study conducted among females, beginning when they were nine years of age. The objective was to examine changes in beverage consumption among these girls and to establish an association between beverage intake, BMI, and nutrient intakes. The beverages studied were milk, regular and diet carbonated sodas, one hundred percent fruit juice, fruit drinks, and coffee/tea. Results show that between childhood and adolescence, carbonated soda intake increases considerably while milk consumption decreases.[39] Over the ten year period, soda consumption nearly tripled, making it the beverage of choice; milk intake, on the other hand, fell by more than twenty-five percent. This shift resulted in a greater intake of calories, higher BMIs, and lower calcium intakes. Consumption of beverages such as fruit-flavored drinks, coffee, and tea also resulted in the ingestion of more sugar and calories, yet less calcium. According to the study's authors, the decline in milk consumption may be partly attributable to the habits of skipping breakfast and eating meals away from home, which become more common during adolescence. Thus, this study confirms the necessity to ensure that kids and teenagers regularly eat healthy, well-balanced breakfasts, routinely participate in family meals at home, and eat out less frequently.

It is well-established that ingesting too many calories leads to weight gain. As previously discussed, regularly drinking sweetened beverages can result in an over-consumption of calories; therefore, a logical conclusion is that frequently drinking sweetened beverages is likely to cause unhealthy weight gain and, consequently, overweight and obesity. Moreover, when considering all of the evidence, there appears to be a strong connection between the ingestion of sweet drinks and the risk of obesity. As a result, decreasing children's and adolescents' sweetened beverage intake is essential for reducing the consumption of excess calories and preventing, as well as reversing, childhood obesity.

Decreased Nutrient Intakes

When a child or adolescent fills up on fluids – including one hundred percent fruit juice – it decreases her appetite for wholesome foods. And as previously mentioned, high-calorie yet low-nutrient sweetened drinks often replace lower-calorie nutrient-dense beverages like milk in the diets of children and adolescents. This typically occurs between the third and eighth grades.[40] However, inadequate milk intake extends to young children as well. Findings from NHANES show that, on average, preschoolers between two and five years old do not meet the recommendations for milk intake.[41] In addition, FITS demonstrates that one hundred percent juice, fruit drinks, and carbonated beverages take the place of milk in toddlers' diets.[42]

Corresponding with the decline in milk consumption, calcium intake among children and adolescents has also fallen.[43,44] Rich in calcium, milk is the primary source of this bone-building mineral in the United States.[45] It is also high in nutrients such as protein, phosphorous, riboflavin, and vitamins A, D, and B_{12}. These nutrients are not usually present in sufficient quantities, or at all, in sweet drinks. It has been found that those who do not consume an adequate amount of milk or dairy products have lower intakes of essential nutrients, including protein.[46] Furthermore, studies show that carbonated beverages in particular are linked to inadequate intakes of calcium, magnesium, phosphorous, riboflavin, vitamin A, and vitamin C among youth.[47,48] It is also worth noting that research demonstrates an association between a higher calcium intake and a lower BMI, even among children and adolescents.[49] Thus, a low calcium intake is particularly undesirable for the prevention and treatment of obesity among youth.

Bone and Oral Health

Because the majority of bone growth occurs during childhood and adolescence, adequate calcium intake is critical during this time. Adolescence is an especially crucial period for the accumulation of bone mass, and insufficient calcium intake can increase the risk of osteoporosis.[50,51] Therefore, it is a serious health concern that milk intake decreases in favor of sweetened beverages as children get older, most significantly among teenagers. Moreover, inadequate calcium intake likely contributes to a greater chance of bone fractures. For example, research has found that compared to adolescent females who do not drink carbonated beverages, those that regularly consume carbonated drinks may be as much as three times more likely to experience a broken bone.[52] Beyond that, multiple studies reveal that cola drinks are associated with a lower bone mineral density and the occurrence of bone fractures.[53] In addition, the large amounts of sugar and acid present in sweetened beverages can adversely affect oral health by causing cavities and the erosion of tooth enamel.[54]

Type 2 Diabetes

According to the Nurses' Health Study II, composed of over one hundred and sixteen thousand female nurses, the frequent consumption of sweetened beverages (carbonated drinks and fruit punch) not only results in a greater intake of calories, weight gain, and a higher BMI, but may also be linked to an increased risk of type 2 diabetes.[55] The greater chance of diabetes remained even after adjusting for other potential risk factors, such as age, physical activity level, and family history of diabetes. The increased diabetes risk is believed to be partly related to the fact that sweetened drinks provide excessive calories as well as large amounts of sugars, such as high-fructose corn syrup, which are absorbed quickly by the body. Related to this, sweet beverages contribute to a high glycemic load, which can cause difficulties with blood sugar control. Conversely, study subjects who reduced their sweetened beverage consumption experienced a significantly lower intake of calories, the least amount of weight gain, and the smallest increases in BMI levels.

Fruit Juice

The American Academy of Pediatrics (AAP) reports that fruit juice is consumed primarily by children, especially those under the age of twelve.[56] For instance, most infants drink an average of two ounces of juice per day juice by the time they turn one year old. However, two percent of infants drink over sixteen ounces per day, while one percent consumes more than twenty-one ounces each day. Toddlers drink approximately six ounces of juice per day, but one out of ten youngsters between two and three years old ingest over twelve ounces each day.[57] Adolescents drink the least amount of juice, probably because they consume more carbonated sodas and fruit-flavored drinks instead.

Results are mixed as to whether or not one hundred percent fruit juice is related to unnecessary weight gain and the development of overweight and obesity. Some studies have found that excessive juice consumption does contribute to unhealthy weight gain and the incidence of overweight, yet others have found that it does not.[58,59] In practice, I often observe the consumption of large amounts of fruit juice among my overweight patients, especially toddlers and young children. Regardless, although one hundred percent fruit juice does not contain any added sweeteners, it is high in natural sugar and tastes very sweet. The underlying principle is that parents and caregivers cannot allow children to develop a habit of regularly ingesting sweet items, especially fluids that go down so easily yet provide little satiety or nutritional value.

Juice Recommendations from the American Academy of Pediatrics

A Policy Statement issued by the AAP provides detailed background information and specific recommendations regarding the consumption of fruit juice among children and adolescents. The Statement indicates that there is no health benefit to consuming one hundred percent fruit juice instead of whole fruit.[60] For example, juice does not contain the fiber that whole fruit does. The AAP also identifies some of the negative effects that can occur when infants and children drink excessive amounts of juice: malnutrition, stunted growth, dental cavities, abdominal discomfort, diarrhea, increased calorie intake, and obesity. The Policy Statement specifies that permitting children to regularly consume juice rather than fruit does not promote positive eating habits, such as that of eating whole fruit. In other words, regularly drinking juice instead of eating fruit is a not a good practice, and allowing children to routinely do so can cause them to establish unhealthy eating habits. Hence, the best choice is to serve children whole fruit rather than juice.

The AAP recommends that fruit juice be limited to four to six ounces per day in younger children between the ages of one and six, and to eight to twelve ounces per day (about two servings) among older children seven to eighteen years of age. [61] Furthermore, the AAP advises that juice not be given to infants younger than six months old, nor served in a baby bottle. Additionally, juice should only be given as part of a meal or snack rather than carried around in a portable cup or container.

According to the AAP, it is easy for toddlers and young children to consume excessive amounts of juice and fruit drinks.[62] This is true for myriad reasons: they taste good (primarily because they are sweet), because they are liquid they can be ingested quickly and easily, and they come in convenient packaging or are poured into a bottle or spill-proof cup to be carried around and sucked on throughout the day. What is more, parents often believe that fruit juice is healthy, so no limits are set. But just as with soda and other sweetened beverages, drinking large amounts of juice can lead to an excessive sugar and calorie intake.

Regardless of what study findings may or may not prove, it is prudent to at least abide by the American Academy of Pediatrics' recommendations and limit the amount of juice that is served to children, if any is offered at all. For starters, serve only one hundred percent fruit juice (ensure that no sugar, corn syrup, or other sweeteners are added) in small amounts in a cup. On top of that, dilute juice with water, especially for younger children, in order to reduce the sugar content and sweetness.

I am stricter than the AAP with my juice recommendations. Personally, except for rare special occasions, I do not offer juice to my children. My professional recommendation is to avoid serving juice to infants under one year of age. For young children, I recommend no more than two to four ounces (one-fourth to one-half cup) of juice per day, mixed at least half-and-half with water; diluted, this provides a total of four to eight ounces to drink. For school-aged children, four to six ounces (one-half to three-quarters cup) is appropriate, preferably diluted with some water. Children meet their entire vitamin C requirement with a four ounce (one-half cup) serving – or less – of one hundred percent fruit juice, so drinking more than this is essentially the same as drinking sugar water, because excess juice provides nothing but sugar and empty calories.

In the cases of obese children and adolescents, or those that are at-risk, recommendations regarding juice intake should be more individualized. Begin with assessing the amount of juice currently being consumed. If a child or teenager is attached to his juice, he can gradually cut back until he is drinking an amount that is within recommendations, or none at all; if the child is younger, also begin diluting the juice with water. If he is not attached to his juice, he can quit drinking it altogether or immediately cut back to an amount that is within guidelines. However, if weight is an issue with your child or adolescent, please consult a registered dietitian with experience in pediatric obesity because recommendations need to be tailored to your child.

Although sports drinks are lower in sugar and calories than other sweetened beverages, they are designed to be used by athletes during competition as a source of carbohydrates for energy, to replace electrolytes lost in sweat, and for hydration. Consequently, these drinks not only contain sugar and calories, but they are relatively high in sodium; thus, it is not appropriate for an average child or adolescent to regularly consume sports drinks.

The low-calorie flavored waters manufactured for children contain alternative sweeteners, such as acesulfame potassium and/or sucralose, which are inappropriate for children to ingest on a regular basis. It varies depending upon the brand, but some also contain high fructose corn syrup, sugar, and calories, but zero nutritional value. Others do contain some juice and provide vitamin C. But they all taste (unnaturally) sweet.

Please refer to "The Truth about Juice" section in chapter four for additional information regarding juice.

Milk

When counseling overweight children and their families, it is not uncommon to discover that an over-consumption of milk is part of the problem. Toddlers and young children, in particular, frequently drink large amounts of whole milk because youngsters between one and two years of age require this high-fat milk for brain development. Oftentimes, however, parents do not switch to lower-fat milk after a child's second birthday. One study found that fewer than nine percent of two to five year olds drink low-fat or non-fat milk rather than whole milk, even though low-fat or non-fat milk is recommended for most children over the age of two.[63] In many cases, a toddler has yet to be completely weaned from the bottle, so she drinks bottles full of milk throughout the day. And many times toddlers that have been weaned from the bottle are attached to some type of spill-proof toddler cup, so they carry around cups full of milk all day long. Just as with juice, it is imperative to ensure that toddlers and young children do not run around with bottles or cups full of milk to sip on at their leisure.

There are a several remedies to this problem. First, toddlers need to be weaned to a cup as soon after their first birthday as possible because children naturally drink less from a cup than from the bottle. Secondly, milk needs to be served in small amounts (about four to six ounces for younger children, up to eight ounces for older children and adolescents) with meals and snacks; only water should be offered to drink between meal- and snack times. Furthermore, toddlers should transition from whole milk to lower-fat milk on their second birthday, unless otherwise directed by a registered dietitian or doctor.

Among school-aged children and adolescents, the consumption of flavored milk containing added sugar, such as chocolate or strawberry milk, often becomes an issue. However, an excessive intake of any type of milk can lead to the consumption of too many calories and unhealthy weight gain. If a child eats plenty of dairy products like yogurt and cheese throughout the day, he may not need to drink much (or any) milk; remember to count the milk that is poured over your child's breakfast cereal towards his daily dairy intake. On the other hand, if a child over the age of two does not consume an adequate amount of dairy or calcium-containing dairy alternatives, he should drink an age-appropriate serving of low-fat

(1%) or non-fat (skim) milk or a calcium-fortified milk substitute with meals and/or snacks in order to meet recommendations.

Recommendations for Dairy Product Intake

According to the *2010 Dietary Guidelines for Americans*, children between two and eight years of age require a total of sixteen to twenty ounces (two to two-and-a-half cups) of dairy products per day.[64] Because young children eat small servings, they usually consume about four to six ounces (one-half to three-quarters cup) of milk or yogurt, or approximately one ounce of natural cheese (equivalent to a six ounce or three-quarters cup serving of dairy), at a time. Therefore, these youngsters typically need about three to four small servings of dairy products each day. Older children and adolescents require a total of twenty-four ounces (three cups) of dairy per day, and a serving size is equivalent to one cup (eight ounces) of milk or yogurt, or one-and-a-half ounces of natural cheese. As a result, older children and adolescents usually need to consume dairy products about three times a day.

Comparison of Sugar and Calories in Beverages and Desserts

The following chart compares the amount of sugar and calories present in some common beverages, including fruit juice and milk, to one another and to various sweet dessert items. Bear in mind, the numbers listed indicate the amount of sugar and calories present in eight fluid ounces; in reality, an individual container of a specific product may contain more or less than this amount. Please also note that all of the numbers are approximations. For example, virtually identical products manufactured by different companies may vary in their sugar and calorie contents, and various flavors or product types among the same brand are likely to contain differing amounts of sugar and calories. To provide a visual, one teaspoon of sugar is equivalent to one sugar cube. As you review this table, notice that one hundred percent fruit juice contains virtually the same amount of sugar and calories as regular soda. The same is true for flavored milks and sweet desserts.

Comparison of Sugar and Calories in Various Non-Diet Beverages and Sweet Desserts*

Beverage	Grams of Sugar in 8 Ounces	Teaspoons of Sugar (and Number of Sugar Cubes) in 8 Ounces	Number of Calories in 8 Ounces
Plain Water	0	0	0
Regular Cola	27	7	100
Regular Lemon-Lime Soda	25	6	100
Regular Orange Soda	33	8	127
100% Apple Juice	26	6.5	110
100% Grape Juice	36	9	140
100% Orange Juice	22	5.5	110
Original Capri Sun®	21	5	80
100% Juice Capri Sun®	27	7	107
Energy Drink	29	7	110
Sports Drink	14	3.5	50
Lemonade	28	7	110
Fruit Punch	25	6	90
Iced Tea	23	6	80
Bottled Coffee Drinks	26	6.5	152
Plain Low-fat (1%) Milk	12	3	110
Low-fat Chocolate Milk	28	7	170
Low-fat Strawberry Milk	30	7.5	180

Sweet Desserts	Grams of Sugar in 8 Ounces	Teaspoons of Sugar (and Number of Sugar Cubes) in 8 Ounces	Number of Calories in 8 Ounces
Jelly Beans (14 pieces)	30	7.5	150
Cotton Candy (1 ounce)	28	7	110
Gummy Bears (14 pieces)	23	6	130
Fudgesicle® (1 bar, 65 grams)	14	3.5	100
Chocolate Ice Cream (1/2 cup)	15	4	140
Candy Bar (1 standard bar, approximately 60 grams)	30	7.5	Not applicable**
Apple Pie (1 slice, approximately 125 grams)	20	5	Not applicable**
Fudge Brownie (1 square, approximately 28 grams)	16	4	170
Chocolate Chip Cookies (1 serving, approximately 33 grams)	11	3	160

* Product ingredients, formulations, and nutrition information may change. Please refer to current product packaging for the most accurate and up-to-date nutrition facts.

** Calorie content is extraordinarily high due to a high fat content, which is not the case with sweetened beverages or the other sweets listed.

Beverage Intake Recommendations

To ascertain your child's beverage intake, ask. "How much plain water did my child drink today? What amount of plain milk and how much flavored milk did he or she consume? What was the amount of one hundred percent fruit juice? How many other sweetened beverages, like soda, fruit-flavored drinks, or lemonade, did my child have?" The answers to these questions will help you determine if any modifications need to be made to your child's beverage consumption.

Current research reveals that decreasing the intake of high-calorie, low-nutrient beverages will likely aid in preventing and reversing childhood and adolescent obesity.[65] In addition, according to FITS, parents and caregivers must not permit children to drink large amounts of any beverage, including milk and one hundred percent fruit juice, because they may take the place of other foods in the diet, as well as lead to an excessive calorie intake.[66]

In general, water should be the thirst-quencher of choice among children and adolescents. Caffeine-free herbal teas without added sugar or other sweeteners are also an option. Fruit juice and sweetened beverages are acceptable once in a while, such as on a special occasion, but when they are a daily habit, sweet drinks can become a problem. Even occasionally, these beverages should be consumed in moderate amounts, such as six to twelve ounces, rather than from enormous, over-sized containers. Sugar-free diet beverages containing alternative sweeteners may be an option to consider for adolescents who are overweight or at-risk of becoming so, however, these should not be consumed regularly or in large amounts.

How do we implement changes when it comes to limiting the amount of sweetened beverages children and adolescents consume? First of all, availability at home should be very limited, if at all. As stated in chapter six, "Wholesome Lunches and Snacks," research suggests that kids and teenagers obtain most of their beverages at home. Next, every adult in a child's life needs to strongly encourage and promote the consumption of plain water rather than sweetened beverages. Among all age groups, the types and amounts of drinks being consumed should be closely monitored by parents and caregivers. For older children and adolescents, limits regarding the intake of sweetened beverages both at home and elsewhere should be discussed and agreed upon, with an explanation given as to why. If a child or adolescent already has a weight issue, there is an even greater need to vigilant about her beverage intake, particularly if she drinks them regularly and/or in large quantities. As in all areas, recommendations need to be individualized, and a registered dietitian with knowledge in this area is essential.

There is more to the puzzle: It is not just the modern-day diet that is putting current and future generations at high risk for developing obesity and chronic disease. Inadequate levels of physical activity are another key factor in the rising rates of obesity and serious medical conditions among youngsters. The next chapter discusses this very fact and introduces strategies for combating the problem.

9 ESTABLISHING PHYSICAL ACTIVITY HABITS EARLY

Jamal attends middle school where he is enrolled in a physical education (PE) class this semester. However, the amount of vigorous activity he gets in class is extremely limited. But because he is in PE, his parents have become very lax about encouraging him to be physically active at home. Jamal does not participate in any organized sports. When he gets home from school, he does his homework and then sits in front of the television or computer, typically playing video games. Rather than walking to and from school each day, his mom drops him off and picks him up out in front. On weekends, Jamal usually wants to stay inside and watch TV or play video games rather than go outside and ride bikes or play basketball with his friends. Over time, this lack of daily physical activity is taking its toll on Jamal's body. Although he is not technically overweight yet, his mother and father notice that he is becoming heavier than normal and seems lethargic. In addition, Jamal complains that he does not feel good overall and that he has less energy than he did last year.

Inadequate amounts of physical activity are undoubtedly linked to the development of overweight and obesity in adults, and this connection is true for children and adolescents as well. Over the past few decades, decreasing levels of physical activity have correlated with the growing rates of obesity among all age groups in this nation. Adding to the problem, Americans – particularly children and adolescents – have become more sedentary than ever before.[1,2]

Inadequate Rates of Physical Activity in America

Americans today have developed a dangerously sedentary lifestyle. Approximately half of the adults in the United States do not meet the recommendations for physical activity, with nearly one-quarter taking part in no physical activity at all.[3] Unfortunately, this habit has been passed on to our youngsters. Children are generally inactive for the majority of the day and, on average, spend very little time engaged in vigorous activity – as little as twelve minutes per day.[4] More than sixty percent of children between nine and thirteen years of age are not involved in any organized physical activities outside of the school day, and close to one quarter do not participate in unstructured exercise apart from school, like running around and playing outside.[5] Furthermore, almost three-quarters of ninth through twelfth grade students do not get an adequate amount of activity, with nearly one-fourth taking part in virtually no physical activity during the week.[6] This is unacceptable considering that regular exercise reduces children's and adolescents' likelihood of developing obesity and chronic disease.[7]

Factors Contributing to Decreased Physical Activity

"Screen Time"

A primary reason for the increase in sedentary behaviors among Americans is the dramatic rise in "screen time" usage: the amount of time spent in front of the television, computers, video games, smart phones, and tablets. This is discussed in detail in the following chapter, "Too Much Screen Time."

Family Leisure-Time Activities

Because many parents work full-time (or more) and families tend to be overscheduled, children are spending less time interacting with their families while enjoying non-sedentary leisure-time activities than in the past. For instance, one family came to me seeking guidance for their entire family because they were all overweight. The oldest daughter, severely obese at the age of thirteen, did not know how to ride a bike. Thus, her younger sister, eleven years old and significantly overweight, did not ride a bike either. Needless to say, this family could not go on bike rides together, which would have been beneficial for all of them. Had the parents taken the time to emphasize the importance of physical activity, including teaching their daughters how to ride bikes, they would have had a family activity that they could all enjoy; just as important, this would have helped them stay healthy and physically fit. It is imperative that families spend time being physically active purely for the sake of enjoyment and having fun together.

Walking to School

Unlike past generations, today's children rarely walk to school or the bus stop. This is often related to safety concerns, but this opportunity for exercise need not be abandoned altogether. When I was young, my parents would respond to my complaints about walking to school or the bus stop by explaining that they had to "walk miles to school". . . "uphill both ways" . . . "even in the snow." I used to question the validity of their replies, but now I am convinced that they were not exaggerating. Back in their day, it was not normal for parents to chauffer their kids to and from school. Even the availability of a family vehicle was much different than it is today – a family may have owned a car, but Father usually took it to work for the day. Plus, it was generally safer for kids to walk longer distances without an adult. The outcome of their lifestyle was a positive one: previous generations did not face the issue of childhood obesity and disease like we do today.

Modernization

Ultimately, some of the causes of inadequate physical activity in our nation are beyond our control, but that does not mean that we give up; there are alternatives, as will be discussed at the end of this chapter. For example, the sizes of yards in newly-built neighborhoods are shrinking, leaving little space for kids to go outside and play in the safety of their own backyard. Furthermore, because of safety concerns, parents now schedule "play dates" for children rather than having all of the kids in the neighborhood get together to run around and play outside. Moreover, urbanization has led to a reduction in physical activity by eliminating or decreasing the amount of time spent in activities of daily living, such as doing chores around the house or walking to school.[8] Urban development has also contributed to a lack of sidewalks, bike paths, and safe recreational facilities (like playgrounds and basketball courts) in communities and neighborhoods.[9]

Technological Advances

Technological advances have caused society to become more "mechanized"; as a result, we are involved in less physical labor on a day-to-day basis. At work, many individuals are completely inactive, sitting at a desk for hour upon hour. At home, we can shop on-line from our personal computer for practically anything, and purchases are delivered right to our front door. We own machines and gadgets that can do whatever we need with very little effort, from automatically opening cans to slicing hard-boiled eggs to opening jars. Americans have come to rely on motorized transportation, as opposed to walking or riding a bike, more than any other country or time in history. And there is the all-important remote control that saves us from having to get up and down to change the TV channel or turn on the lights or close the blinds – a remote control is available for virtually anything we need to do. Our culture's desire for convenience has resulted in the expenditure of fewer calories each day with the consequence of unhealthy weight gain.

Physical Activity at School

Although we cannot entirely depend upon the school system to provide children with the physical activity they need, schools are an important component to the physical health of children simply because they spend so much time there. Unfortunately, opportunities for exercise at school have diminished over the years. Significant changes in the availability and requirements of physical education (PE) programs and recess have resulted in less physical activity among students.[10] For instance, attendance of a daily PE class among high school students dropped from approximately forty-two percent in 1991 to thirty-three percent in 2009.[11] In 2006, less than thirty-nine percent of school districts examined as part of the School Health Policies and Programs Study (led by the Centers for Disease Control and Prevention) recommended at least thirty minutes of recess at the elementary school level each day.[12]

Physical education classes, as well as some extracurricular sports and physical activities, have long been considered less important than academic subjects, thus they are often among the first programs to receive cut-backs or be eliminated by school districts. And even when PE classes or extracurricular physical activities are offered, large class sizes or lack of equipment may result in insufficient programs.[13]

What is more, the recommendations given by The National Association of State Boards of Education for one hundred and fifty minutes of physical education per week for elementary students and two hundred and twenty-five minutes per week for middle and high school students are not being met.[14] In a study conducted among third-graders at ten different locations, students spent thirty-three minutes twice a week in PE, with only twenty-five minutes per week at a moderate or vigorous intensity level.[15] Furthermore, very few schools provided daily physical education for all students in 2006: less than four percent of elementary schools, approximately eight percent of middle schools, and about two percent of high schools.[16] However, whether or not schools offer appropriate amounts of physical activity for kids, it is critical that parents and caregivers encourage and provide opportunities for plenty of exercise at home.

Benefits of Regular Physical Activity

There are countless positive outcomes to being physically active on a regular basis. The benefits for adults are undisputed. Exercise aids in weight loss and weight management; blood sugar control; blood pressure regulation; enhancing psychological and emotional well-being; and reducing the risk of chronic diseases such as heart disease, stroke, type 2 diabetes, certain cancers (such as colon and breast cancer), and osteoporosis.[17,18] In addition, regular activity strengthens bones, muscles, and joints; reduces anxiety and depression; and improves sleep.[19,20] Many individuals use exercise as a stress reliever. A medical doctor once admitted to me during her residency that if she did not jog every evening after work, she probably would have needed a prescription for an anti-anxiety or anti-depressant medication. Possibly most convincing, for every hour spent engaging in regular exercise, you can increase your life expectancy by about two hours.[21]

Children and Adolescents

The numerous advantages of physical activity extend to children and adolescents as well.[22,23] Research has established a strong correlation between lack of physical activity and the risk of obesity among children and adolescents. For example, one analysis reveals that obese children spend less time being moderately and/or vigorously active than those who are not obese.[24] Findings from a National Health and Nutrition Examination Survey demonstrate that children who exert the least amount of energy in physical activity and/or spend the most time watching television tend to be the most overweight.[25] The compelling Stanford GEMS (Girls health Enrichment Multi-site Studies) pilot examined the potential of an after-school dance class coupled with decreased television usage (including videos and video games) in reducing unhealthy weight gain among low-income eight to ten year old African-American girls. The results show a trend towards healthier body weights, increased physical activity levels, significantly less television usage among the girls and their families, and fewer dinners eaten while watching TV.[26] Additionally, the girls exhibited fewer concerns about weight and a tendency towards better grades in school. Not only are less active children more likely to be overweight, but they have a higher risk of high blood pressure, elevated cholesterol and insulin levels, and abnormal lipid (blood fat) values, which can lead to serious health problems.[27] What is more, regular physical activity leads to improved self-esteem and overall self-image among youth, regardless of their weight status.[28]

A Two-Pronged Approach

Weight loss/maintenance and disease prevention require a two-pronged approach. Healthy eating and physical activity are both essential for promoting health and well-being; these two elements go hand in hand. I like to use the illustration of a balance scale. A person may eat healthy, but if they neglect to exercise regularly, their health will be out of balance (please refer to Figure 1). On the other hand, a person may engage in plenty of physical activity, but if they have a terrible diet, they will be unbalanced (refer to Figure 2). However, if a person routinely eats right and gets an adequate amount of exercise, their body will be in balance, they will be able to manage their weight, and they will decrease their risk of chronic disease (refer to Figure 3).

Figure 1: Healthy Eating and Inadequate Physical Activity

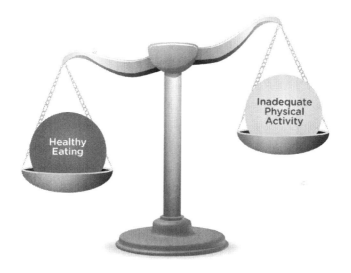

Figure 2: Unhealthy Eating and Adequate Physical Activity

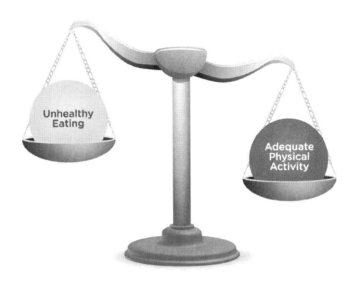

Figure 3: Healthy Eating and Physical Activity in Balance

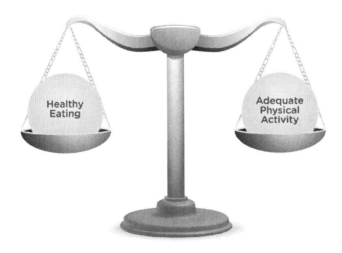

Establishing Physical Activity Habits Early

According to the Centers for Disease Control and Prevention, "Childhood and adolescence may be pivotal times for developing the habit of regular physical activity and preventing sedentary behavior among adults. Positive experiences with physical activity at a young age help lay the basis for being regularly active throughout life."[29] In other words, engaging in physical activity during childhood and adolescence influences an individual's exercise habits in adulthood.[30]

It is imperative that parents and caregivers shift our mindsets regarding physical activity, which will in turn serve to change our children's attitudes about being active. Rather than seeing exercise as a duty or an obligation – as something we "have" to do, adults must learn to view it as something that is fun and enjoyable – as something we like to do. Then kids will start to do the same.

As emphasized in chapter four, early habits are likely to become lifelong habits. As such, it is crucial to start encouraging children to be active (and discouraging inactivity) when they are very young – as early as infancy and toddlerhood. In fact, physical activity habits may become established as early as the preschool years, at about two to five years of age.[31] As with healthy eating, getting an adequate amount of exercise is not only important for the short-term, immediate benefits, but it is also vital in the long-term for a child's future health and well-being. In fact, it may be just as important to a toddler's overall health as the eating habits she is forming. When young ones are physically active on a regular basis, it leads to the development of a routine that will continue as they get older, ideally for a lifetime.

Parents and caregivers cannot expect children to turn off the television, video game, or computer and be excited to go outside and play if we do not instill this habit early on. And it will only become more of an issue as they grow older because as children move from childhood into adolescence and adulthood, they tend to become less physically active.[32,33] A main point of this book is that if parents and caregivers allow babies, toddlers, and young children to engage in sedentary behaviors such as watching TV and videos or playing video games rather than getting an adequate amount of physical activity every day, children are going to want to continue this habit as they get older. And a pattern of inactivity contributes to the development of obesity and adverse health conditions, such as heart disease and diabetes.

It may be surprising, but even babies and toddlers need to be active on a regular basis as well as limit sedentary activities. There are many ways to encourage little ones to move: dance to children's music, march around the room, do stretches on the floor, play various active and movement games, allow your child to "explore" in a safe environment, play "chase" or a version of "tag" around the house or outside, go for a walk or tricycle ride around the neighborhood, walk to the park (or just go play at a park), run around and play in the backyard together, or take him to a toddler gym or other type of open gym. A game of "Hide-and-Seek" is fun for children of all ages; another favorite is "Duck, Duck, Goose!" And it is not difficult to incorporate more movement into various games or activities. For instance, in "Duck, Duck, Goose!," run around the house rather than just around the circle. Additional activities that incorporate movement include digging with plastic shovels, cups, and buckets; playing dress-up with hats, shoes, dresses, and other items; and acting out stories from your favorite books together. It is essential to teach growing babies and young children that being physically active is an important and fun habit.

Recommendations for Physical Activity

Adults

According to the *2008 Physical Activity Guidelines for Americans,* adults eighteen to sixty-four years old should engage in at least one-hundred and fifty minutes (two-and-a-half hours) of moderate aerobic activity, such as walking briskly, or seventy-five minutes (one hour and fifteen minutes) of vigorous aerobic exercise, like jogging, each week – or an equal combination thereof.[34] For greater health benefits, it is recommended that adults increase their weekly aerobic activity to three-hundred minutes (five hours) of moderate aerobic exercise or one-hundred and fifty minutes (two-and-a-half hours) of vigorous aerobic activity, or an equivalent combination. The *Guidelines* also state that there are further health advantages to participating in additional amounts of physical activity. It is specified that aerobic exercise should be completed in periods lasting at least ten minutes, as well as be spread evenly throughout the week. In addition, the *Guidelines* advise adults to engage in exercises that will strengthen all major muscles groups, such as sit-ups, push-ups, and lifting weights, at least two days per week.

The physical activity guidelines issued by the American College of Sports Medicine (ACSM) in 2007 are similar to the *2008 Physical Activity Guidelines for Americans.* For healthy adults between the ages of eighteen and sixty-five to maintain health and reduce the risk of chronic disease, the ACSM recommends engaging in moderately-intense cardiovascular activity for a minimum of thirty minutes per day, five days a week or vigorously-intense cardiovascular exercise for at least twenty minutes a day, three days per week, or an equivalent combination of both.[35] However, to lose weight or maintain weight loss, they state that sixty to ninety minute periods of moderate intensity aerobic exercise on most days of the week may be necessary. In addition, the ACSM advises performing strength-training exercises two times per week.

While the various guidelines may seem overwhelming and confusing, that should not be a deterrent from exercising altogether. My general recommendation for adults who are not currently active on a regular basis is to gradually increase your physical activity level, with the goal of eventually reaching a recommended amount of exercise; any activity beyond what you are currently doing is beneficial. For example, start with just thirty minutes, two times per week. Gradually work up to three to four times per week, then increase to at least forty-five minutes per session. An achievable final goal is forty-five minutes to one hour, four to five times per week. This should include both cardiovascular (aerobic) exercise as well as strength-training. In addition, vary the types of exercise you engage in – if you perform the same routine day after day, your body will eventually become accustomed to it and your fitness level will plateau. At the same time, ensure that you enjoy what you are doing or you will not continue it long-term. If you find that you have the time and can benefit from additional amounts of activity, seventy-five to ninety minutes (one hour and fifteen minutes to one-and-a-half hours), four to five times a week is a good goal; be sure to give your body at least two days per week, preferably not in a row, to rest and recover.

Children and Adolescents

The *2008 Physical Activity Guidelines for Americans* recommend that children and adolescents six to seventeen years of age participate in at least sixty minutes (one hour) of physical activity every day.[36] This guideline is delineated into three categories of activity: aerobic, muscle-strengthening, and bone-strengthening. The majority of the sixty minutes per day should be comprised of moderately- or vigorously-intense aerobic activity, with vigorously-intense activity occurring at least three days per week. Aerobic activities include running, hopping, skipping, jumping rope, swimming, dancing, and bicycling.

In addition, as part of their sixty minutes of daily activity, children and adolescents should engage in muscle-strengthening activities three or more days a week. Such activities include playing on playground equipment, climbing trees, and playing tug-of-war. For older children and teenagers, muscle-strengthening exercises may be more structured, such as using resistance bands or lifting weights, assuming that qualified supervision is provided and appropriate technique is used.

And last, children and adolescents should participate in bone-strengthening activities at least three days each week, which counts toward their weekly physical activity quota. Bone-strengthening activities consist of any movement that puts force upon the bones, which promotes bone growth and strength. Examples include running, jumping rope, basketball, tennis, or hopscotch, in which force is produced by impact with the ground. As the examples demonstrate, bone-strengthening exercises may also be aerobic or muscle-strengthening activities.

The *Guidelines* specify that any amount of appropriate physical activity done by children and adolescents, regardless of how brief, counts toward the daily total of sixty minutes.[37] The *Guidelines* emphasize the importance of enabling children and adolescents to take part in activities that are developmentally- and age-appropriate, enjoyable, and varied. It is also essential to encourage children to participate in activities that they enjoy and, as often as possible, that they can do along with family or friends. Adolescents, especially, are strongly influenced by their peers, so helping them choose activities that they like and that include their friends is critical.

Again, these recommendations can appear complex and cumbersome. To simplify, a good general goal for children and adolescents is to be physically active at least one hour per day, at least five days per week while at the same time strictly limiting "screen time," which will be specifically addressed in the following chapter. Ensuring that children and teenagers participate in some type of vigorous activity at least a few times per week is also prudent.

Young Children

While the *2008 Physical Activity Guidelines* do not give specific recommendations for children between two and five years of age, experts agree that young children should engage in active play several times each day.[38] The American Heart Association recommends that toddlers and preschoolers spend at least one hour playing actively each day, as well as limited time in sedentary activities, such as watching television.[39]

Tips for Increasing Physical Activity among Children and Adolescents

Start by assessing your child's physical fitness level, which is not difficult to do. Can he run up the stairs without becoming winded? At the playground, is she running around and playing or is she sitting on the side with a handheld video game or smartphone? How often does he go outside and play or ride bikes rather than sit in front of a screen? Is she involved in any organized sports or activity programs after school hours or on the weekends? Does your family get out and be active together on a regular – at least weekly – basis? Once you have determined your family's current level of physical activity, you can begin working to improve it.

- Be active together as a family. Go for a walk, hike, or bike ride; go swimming, rollerblading, roller skating, ice skating, or to the park. Play Frisbee®, volleyball, badminton, tennis, racquetball, or basketball. Go bowling, fishing, golfing, or play a round of miniature golf.

- Have a picnic and then play catch or fly kites afterwards.

- Turn on the music and dance! Children and teenagers of all ages love to listen and move to music.

- Take a family trip to the zoo, aquarium, nature conservancy, wildlife refuge, botanical gardens, or arboretum. These destinations often have trails for walking or hiking, providing an ideal "exercise" opportunity for the entire family.

- When the weather permits, go to the beach or lakefront and run around and play in the sand and water. Simply digging in the sand and building sandcastles exerts energy.

- Encourage your child to get outside and play – whether in your backyard, in her friend's or neighbor's backyard, or by taking her to play at the park.

- Walk your child to school or the bus stop; or ride bikes or non-motorized scooters to get there. Compared to children who are driven, studies have found that students who walk or bicycle to school tend to have higher overall activity levels.[40,41] And it is perfect exercise for the rest of the family, too.

- Activities such as playing hopscotch, jumping rope with friends, dancing, climbing, riding bikes, skating or rollerblading, walking the dog, doing yard work or gardening with the family, washing the car, training during the off-season, or structured weight-lifting may be more readily accepted by children or adolescents than simply recommending that they get involved in organized sports or "go exercise."[42]

- When it is warm outside, set up a sprinkler and run, jump, and play as a family.

- When the weather does not allow for outdoor activities, initiate indoor activities rather than sitting in front of the television or computer. There are many books available at the library filled with rainy-day activity ideas. Even if it is not "exercise," anything is better than spending hours in front of a screen. For instance, going to the library is better than being sedentary at home.

- Be creative! Use your imagination and your kids' imaginations to come up with fun, unique ideas that work for your family. In their book, *What Every Child Needs*, Elisa Morgan and Carol Kuykendall explain ways to make exercise fun: "Jumping rope and jumping jacks to music are two fun exercises. Children can also create their own Olympics or triathlons. Exercising can be fun, and learning that now helps children grow up to be healthy adults."[43]

- Build your own family-friendly obstacle course, indoors or outside.

- Go to the mall if it has an indoor play area. Avoid frequenting play places that serve food, unless you can resist the temptation to make a purchase or will be satisfied to buy something minimal and healthy, such as a small low-fat milk or apple slices.

- Invest time and money in your own health as well as the health of your children. Purchase a family membership to a gym or recreation/community center that caters to both children and adults, such as the YMCA. If something like this is not financially feasible, ask about scholarships that may be available.

- The YMCA serves as a great model for encouraging and fostering physical activity among children of all ages and their families. The Y has physical activity programs available for children as early as infancy, such as parent-child swim and toddler gym classes. They offer dance, gymnastics, and sports programs for children beginning as early as three years of age. The YMCA also has a variety of sports programs and other activities for older children and teenagers. Many other gyms offer similar programs. What a great way to instill healthy habits and a love for being active!

- Get your child involved in one of the various programs or activities offered by your local parks and recreation department. If you are unfamiliar with their programs, look through one of the catalogs they publish (often available on-line), and you will be amazed at the multitude of activities they offer.

- Is your child interested in taking dance classes, swimming lessons, gymnastics, or horseback riding lessons? How about looking into ice skating lessons, ice hockey, or tennis or golf lessons?

- Sign your child up for an organized/recreational sports program, such as basketball, baseball, soccer, or volleyball, whether through the local parks and recreation department, community center, YMCA, or local gym. Research what is available near you and you will find that almost all sports are represented by one organization or another.

- If your child is interested, enroll him in a martial arts program, such as Tae Kwon Do. Not only will your child be physically active, it may help his performance at school and aid in the development of social skills; martial arts programs have been associated with improvements in self-control, classroom conduct, and socialization, especially among boys.[44]

- Park further away from your destination, such as the store or doctor's office, so that you have to walk farther to get there – every step you make throughout the day counts. Also, use the stairs rather than the escalator or elevator whenever possible. Turn these into habits that you do all the time – both with your family as well as when you are on your own. Your children will then adopt these habits as their own.

- For more ideas, refer to the "Screen Time Alternatives" section at the end of the following chapter, "Too Much Screen Time."

A primary reason children and adolescents engage in too little physical activity is that they are spending far too much time in front of screens, including the television, video games, and computers. This topic is discussed in the following chapter, along with ways to decrease "screen time."

10 TOO MUCH SCREEN TIME

Ten year old Josefina does not like to go outside and play. Nor does she enjoy reading for pleasure. For that matter, other than the homework she is required to complete, Josefina rarely engages in activities that require her to be active, creative, or simply use her imagination. Josefina prefers to spend her free time playing video games. Whether it is the video game system in their family room, the computer in her bedroom, or the handheld game device that she takes with her practically everywhere she goes – even to the park, Josefina is usually playing a video game of some sort. Over the last couple of years, Josefina's parents have watched her become increasingly "chubby." Though she eats fairly healthfully, they are beginning to realize that Josefina spends virtually all of her free-time completely inactive in front of some type of video game screen. And when she is not playing video games, she typically watches television or surfs the Internet.

Americans are spending more time in front of screens than ever before, and this "screen time" is directly related to the increasing prevalence of obesity in our nation. Screen time usage comprises television (TV), digital video discs (DVDs) and videos, movies, video games, computers, smartphones like an iPhone, and tablets such as an iPad. The average American family today owns three to four TV sets, two to three DVD players or video cassette recorders (VCRs), two video game systems, and two computers.[1] These numbers are significantly higher than in past decades. For example, in 1970 only thirty-five percent of homes had more than one TV and as few as six percent had three (or more) television sets.[2] Further, ownership of novel technological devices, like smartphones and tablets, grows considerably with each passing year.

Older Children and Adolescents

More specifically, media use sky-rocketed among children and adolescents over the course of ten years. From 1999 to 2009, the average amount of time that youth between eight and eighteen years of age spent in front of a screen rose from approximately four hours and forty-five minutes to more than seven hours every day; this is largely due to a greater amount of time spent playing video games and on the computer.[3] On the other hand, this age group only spends about a half-hour of each day reading for pleasure. Thus, the amount of time these kids spend in front of a screen is fourteen times greater than the length of time they spend reading.

Television continues to be the primary source of entertainment among youth eight to eighteen years old, with an average of four-and-a-half hours of TV-viewing per day.[4] The computer occupies an additional one hour and thirty minutes of daily free time while another hour and fifteen minutes is spent playing video games; ten years ago, computer and video games each took up a half-hour of the day, for a combined total of only one hour.[5] Among youth, eleven to fourteen year olds spend the greatest amount of time watching television, at more than five hours per day; this group also spends the most time on the computer and playing video games.[6]

In 1970, only six percent of sixth graders had a TV in their bedroom.[7] Today, almost three-quarters of those between the ages of eight and eighteen have a television in their room; this is compelling because those with a television in their bedroom watch about an hour more of TV per day compared to those without one.[8] Beyond television sets, almost sixty percent of eight to eighteen year olds have a DVD player or VCR in their room, up from just thirty-six percent in 1999; moreover, half have a video game system in their bedroom.[9] These figures do not include portable movie players or handheld video game devices which are becoming commonplace among all age groups. Additionally, more than one-third of youths between eight and eighteen have a computer in their room with virtually the same proportion having Internet access, compared to only one-fifth and one-tenth, respectively, in 1999.

In many homes, there are no limits regarding the amount of television that children and teenagers may view, and it is on for the majority of the day. For instance, nearly half of eight to eighteen year olds report that the TV is on for most of the day in their home, even if no one is watching it.[10] Furthermore, almost two-thirds say that the television is typically on during family mealtimes. Children who live in homes where the TV is left on for a large amount of the day spend significantly more time watching it. As an example, youth from homes where the television is on for most of the day watch an hour-and-a-half more than those who report that the TV is rarely or never on while no one is watching.[11]

Infants, Toddlers, and Young Children

Older children and adolescents are not the only concerns in regards to screen time. Infants, toddlers, and young children are being exposed to too much television and overall screen time as well. Over eighty percent of children six years old and under spend time in front of a screen on a normal day.[12] These young children watch a screen for an average of two hours per day, usually TV and DVDs/videos; this is about the same amount of time they spend playing outside, and triple the amount of time they spend reading.

The American Academy of Pediatrics recommends that children under the age of two be exposed to no television or other screens at all. Regardless of this recommendation, over two-thirds of infants and toddlers less than two years old regularly spend time in front of a screen: about sixty percent watch television, forty-two percent watch DVDs or videos, five percent play on the computer, and three percent play video games; these young ones spend an average of two hours per day in front of a screen.[13] Similarly, a survey conducted among parents of children between two and twenty-four months of age reveals that forty percent of three month old infants regularly watch television or DVDs/videos, and that by the age of two, nine out of ten little ones spend two to three hours in front of the TV each day.[14]

Approximately two-thirds of children six and under live in households where the television is on at least half of the time, even if no one is watching it; more than one-third live in homes where the TV is on most or all of the time.[15] Moreover, almost half of parents report that they are likely to use the TV to occupy their zero to six year old so that they can complete an important task; not surprisingly, these children spend an additional half-hour in front of the television set each day.[16]

Children who live in homes where the television is on all or most of the time are much more likely to watch TV before they turn one year old, to watch TV every day, and to watch for longer periods of time than children who live in households where the television is not on as often.[17] Furthermore, these children are less likely to read every day, and when they do spend time reading, it is for a shorter amount of time. Interestingly, these children are also less likely to be able to read independently. According to parents, fifty-six percent of four to six year olds in homes where the TV is rarely on can read, compared to only thirty-four percent of those in households where the TV is on all or most of the time.

Many toddlers and young children are not just passively sitting in front of screens, but they are actively asking for or helping themselves to the television, DVDs or videos, and the computer.[18] A quarter of children under the age of two and over forty percent of four to six year olds have a TV in their bedroom.[19] In addition, more than one quarter of children between zero and six have a DVD player or VCR in their room, while ten percent have their own video game system. Young children with television sets, DVD players/

VCRs, or video games in their room spend a greater amount of time in front of them compared to those who do not.

A major concern regarding screen time is that it may take the place of other activities in children's lives, such as playing outside or reading. A study by the Kaiser Family Foundation shows that compared to those who watch less television, four to six year olds who watch two or more hours of TV per day spend approximately one half-hour less playing outside as well as fewer minutes reading each day.[20]

The Effects of Television Viewing on Body Weight

Time and time again, research has established a definitive link between a child's weight and her television viewing habits – specifically, the amount of time she spends watching TV. In fact, time spent in front of the television is associated with unhealthy weight gain independent of other factors including diet/caloric intake, physical activity level, race/ethnicity, socioeconomic status, and age.[21,22] Two large studies demonstrate that while the number of overweight individuals in both the United States and England have risen in the last decade, reported caloric and fat intakes have not increased notably in either country.[23] The Health Behaviour in School-Aged Children Study, an international survey conducted in collaboration with the World Health Organization, found that in countries with high rates of childhood and adolescent obesity, overweight youth engage in less physical activity and more television viewing that those who are of normal weight.[24] Additionally, in over ninety percent of the countries studied, reported sugar consumption was actually lower among overweight youth compared to those of normal weight; furthermore, overweight and obesity were not linked to fruit or vegetable intake or soft drink consumption. This evidence proves that sedentary behaviors – namely television viewing and total screen time – and lack of physical activity are major contributors to the obesity epidemic.

The amount of time a child spends watching television correlates to his body fat percentage as well as his body mass index (BMI).[25] Overweight and obesity occur least often among children who watch one hour or less of TV per day, and most often among those who watch four hours or more each day, regardless of age, race/ethnicity, or socioeconomic status.[26] Moreover, research reveals that those with a TV in their bedroom are at greater risk of obesity, even preschoolers.[27]

The overweight children I see for weight-related nutrition counseling typically watch an excessive amount of television each day, and because of the habits they have developed, it is difficult for them to cut their total screen time down to the maximum recommendation of two hours per day. For example, one patient was an obese school-aged child with high cholesterol and triglycerides. He lived in a single-parent home, so he was frequently home alone and spent much of his day in front of a screen. In fact, this child watched television and played video games for about four hours each day. Research and professional experience confirm that children who watch the most TV each day have the highest rates of overweight and obesity, while those who watch the least amount of television tend to have the healthiest BMIs.

Television and Toddlers and Preschoolers

The increased risk of obesity related to too much television extends to toddlers and preschoolers as well. According to the Avon longitudinal study of parents and children, three year olds who watch more than eight hours of television per week (or just over an hour per day) are more likely to be obese at the age of seven.[28] A National Institute of Child Health and Human Development study demonstrates that preschoolers who are *exposed* to TV for two or more hours per day have a greater chance of experiencing obesity; exposure refers to merely being in a room with the television turned on, even if the child is not necessarily watching it.[29] This increased risk is independent of several potential contributing factors, such as the family's socioeconomic status; the mother's marital status, education, age, and symptoms of depression; and the amount of TV exposure that is educational.

Further, researchers who examined the effects of early television usage discovered that TV exposure at the age of two is associated with several consequences at ten years of age: a more sedentary lifestyle, lower levels of physical activity, a greater intake of soft drinks and snacks, a higher BMI, less engagement at school, lower math grades, and more problems with peers.[30] Additionally, television usage at four-and-half years of age is related to risk of negative outcomes at age ten. What is more, the Early Childhood Longitudinal Study (Birth Cohort) shows that watching more than two hours of television (including DVDs and videos) per day increases the risk of obesity among four year olds.[31]

The Connection between Screen Time and Increased Body Weight

The connection between screen time and increased body weight is at least threefold and has both direct and indirect correlations. It was initially believed that the weight gain associated with television viewing was primarily due to the fact it is very passive and takes the place of activities that burn more calories. While this is true, there is also an indirect link between sitting in front of a screen and unhealthy weight gain: when children watch television or use the Internet, they see a plethora of appealing advertisements that promote the consumption of high-calorie foods and beverages. The third correlation is that children tend to eat mindlessly while sitting in front of the TV – typically high-calorie, low-nutrient foods – whether or not they are truly hungry.

Sitting in Front of a Screen Burns Few Calories

First of all, humans burn fewer calories while sitting passively in front of a screen than while doing almost any other activity, including reading. Only sleeping burns fewer calories, and that by just a few. In fact, we may burn more calories doing absolutely nothing than while watching TV. The brain is in its most inactive state when we aimlessly sit and stare at a television or other screen; it is somewhat comparable to being in a comatose state. It would practically be healthier for children to sit and stare at a wall than to watch TV – the brain would be more active because they would be thinking and using their imagination, and as a result, burn more calories. To illustrate this point, we will present some calorie comparisons. The following table is based upon a chart published in the *Harvard Heart Letter*[32] and provides the number of calories a one hundred and twenty-five pound individual would burn while engaged in various activities for a half-hour. Rather than paying attention to the actual number of calories used up for each activity, please note the *relationship* between the amount of calories expended during a half-hour of a certain activity compared to the number of calories burned while watching television for the same amount of time.

Calories Burned During Various Half-Hour Activities

Activity	Calories Burned
Sleeping	19
Watching TV	*23*
Reading while sitting	34
Standing in line	38
Computer work (such as typing, not just sitting and staring at the screen)	41
Sitting in class or meetings	About 50
Cooking/Helping in the kitchen	75
Dancing	90 to 180
Raking the lawn	120
Playing (in general, at a moderate to vigorous activity level)	120 to 150
Washing the car Heavy house cleaning	130
Badminton	135
Gardening	135 to 150
Hopscotch Skateboarding	150
Swimming (in general)	180
Rollerblading	210
Bicycling	255 to 300
Jumping rope	300

As can be surmised from the chart, if hours of television-watching replace more active pursuits, such as playing, dancing, rollerblading, bicycling – even household chores or yard work – the calorie disparity is significant and can add up quickly, causing unhealthy weight gain.

Advertisements for Unhealthy Foods

Children and adolescents view approximately ten food commercials per hour of television they watch; these commercials are usually for fast-food, sweetened breakfast cereals, high-sugar beverages, and sweet treats.[33] This is largely because food manufacturers are targeting children and adolescents. Beyond being fun and entertaining, these advertisements often contain deceptive or incorrect nutrition information.[34] In fact, television watching, including the commercials, is associated with inaccurate nutrition knowledge and poor eating habits among children.[35] As poor discriminators, kids are completely unaware that the sweetened cereal they just saw in the appealing, colorful, loud commercial is detrimental to their health and well-being. When they are in the grocery store and see that product on the shelves, they are going to request it – even beg for it. However, if television viewing is limited at home, children will not see as many misleading commercials for unhealthy foods and beverages; ideally, they will not even be aware that certain products exist and will fail to recognize or request them at the store. Nor will they mistakenly believe that unhealthy items are "good for them."

Research proves that children, even young children, request the items that they see advertised on television. One study found that the total amount of time a child spends watching TV, as well as total screen time overall, is related to her immediate and future requests for the food and beverages she sees in the commercials.[36] Another experiment demonstrates that exposure to thirty-second food commercials during children's programming results in preschoolers selecting the brand of food they see advertised rather than a similar unadvertised item.[37]

Compounding this issue is that food and beverage companies are also marketing their products on the Internet, and they are using a variety of methods to get the attention of children and adolescents.[38] According to researchers, the majority of online advertisements intended to reach children and teenagers are for unhealthy items that could have an adverse effect on their food preferences and selections, as well as their health.[39] In fact, some experts believe that the marketing strategies employed on websites may have more of an influence on youth than do television advertisements.

Eating in Front of the Television

Americans have developed a habit of eating meals and snacks while sitting in front of the television, and this is true for children as well as adults. Indeed, an investigation reveals that children consume more food while watching television (including videos) than while participating in any other activity, including doing homework, reading for pleasure, riding in a vehicle, watching a movie at the theater, or playing.[40]

Both a National Health and Nutrition Examination Survey (NHANES) and the Planet Health intervention and evaluation trial show that the more time a child spends watching TV, the more calories he consumes.[41,42] Many times, children do not pay attention to their hunger and fullness cues while watching television; they may eat even when they are not hungry or continue eating after they have reached the point of satiety. Watching television or playing video games while eating could interfere with the body's ability to sense its internal hunger and fullness signals, leading to overeating.[43] As a matter of fact, preschoolers who are accustomed to eating in front of the TV will eat more while watching television than if it is turned off.[44] Researchers concluded that children who regularly eat while watching television may become insensitive to the biological cues that regulate food intake. This has significant implications.

There are at least a few reasons that children, as well as adults, tend to overeat while watching television. To begin with, they are engrossed in the show they are watching rather than paying attention to the messages that are being transmitted from the stomach to their brain. Thus, they are highly distracted and finish off the entire bag of chips or plate of food that is in front of them without being conscious of how it relates to their hunger and fullness levels. Secondly, it is impossible to socialize while eating in front of the television set. Conversing, laughing, and interacting during a meal require us to eat more slowly, helping us to sense and respond to our hunger and fullness cues. Watching television prevents this from occurring. Last, as described in the preceding section, we are bombarded with food commercials during television viewing. Simply seeing these advertisements gives us the idea – the urge – to eat something. Ponder this, and ask your children to think about it as well: when you go to the pantry or refrigerator after watching a food advertisement on

TV, do you get up for food because you are physiologically hungry or because seeing food on the TV compels you to do so? As originally described in chapter four, "Healthy Eating Habits Begin Early," it is imperative to heed the body's signals of hunger and fullness; this becomes even more crucial when sitting in front of the television.

What is more, the items that children typically consume while watching television are usually high-calorie, high-sugar, high-fat, and/or high-sodium foods rather than healthy choices like fruits and vegetables.[45] When television is viewed during mealtimes, children tend to eat more red meat, pizza, snack foods, and soft drinks, but fewer fruits and vegetables.[46] For example, the school-aged child mentioned previously regularly ate dinner in front of the television; his typical dinner consisted of a can of Chef Boyardee® ravioli or two hot dogs. On weekends and during the summer, he ate a can of SpaghettiOs® for lunch, usually while watching TV. As a result, his intake of fruits and vegetables was poor. Routinely eating highly processed, calorie-dense, low-nutrient foods – as is the commonly the case when children eat during television viewing – leads to the consumption of excess calories and, over time, unhealthy weight gain.

Nearly every patient I have ever worked with regarding weight issues, whether child or adult, had a habit of eating while watching television when they initially came to meet with me. In some cases, it was routinely eating a meal in front of the television; in other cases, it was regularly snacking past fullness while watching TV. But one way or another, the majority of my patients have had a tendency to watch TV and eat at the same time. By contrast, not each of my overweight patients has had a problem with frequent fast-food intake, inadequate amounts of exercise, or consuming large amounts of empty calories such as regular sodas, mochas, or juice. But almost all have had issues with eating in front of the television. This confirms that eating while watching TV is a widespread contributor to the problem of overweight and obesity in America today.

I believe the tendency to eat in front of the TV is partly due to the fact that even though our minds are distracted by the television, they are not one hundred percent occupied. And because we are mentally and physically inactive while sitting on the couch and staring at the screen, our minds and bodies become "bored" and want something to keep us busy and "active." So, the easiest thing to do is eat. I have found that keeping oneself busy and active while watching TV, such as by doing a craft or working on some type of project or hobby, results in a decreased tendency to eat while sitting in front of the television.

Effects of Decreased Screen Time

So, does decreasing the amount of time a child spends in front of a screen really have an effect? The resounding answer is, "Yes, it truly does." Research has proven so. For example, one study examined the effects of reducing the amount of time spent watching TV (including videos) and playing video games, but did not encourage increased amounts of physical activity in place of screen time. Children who reduced their television usage by an average of nine hours per week gained less body fat and were leaner compared to those who did not; in addition, they ate fewer meals in front of the TV and consumed fewer high-fat foods.[47] A similar investigation followed a larger number of children over a longer period of time. The results were essentially the same: children who reduced the amount of time they spent watching TV/videos and playing video games had lower amounts of body fat, and these lower body fat levels were maintained over time.[48]

Additional Risks of Too Much Screen Time

Besides the adverse effects on body weight, there are additional consequences of spending too much time in front of a screen. An article released by the American Academy of Pediatrics identifies high-risk behaviors among older children and adolescents that may be related to too much television: aggressiveness and violence, substance use and abuse, sexual activity, poor body image, and lower school achievement.[49] According to results of a survey that evaluated the link between media exposure and school performance, both the total amount of screen time (TV, movies, and video games) and screen time content (exposure to adult content) are strongly and independently related to poorer performance at school.[50] This association remains true after controlling for other possible factors, such as the child's age, gender, and socioeconomic status; the mother's parenting style; and the child's levels of self-esteem and rebelliousness. Thus, there is much more at stake than our children's weight. Television is detrimental for youth on multiple levels.

There are also concerns regarding the effects that television may have on the development of infants, toddlers, and young children; specific areas of concern include autism, attention problems, and delayed language development. For instance, researchers have identified a strong correlation between television viewing by children less than three years of age and rates of autism.[51] This is not to imply that watching television at a young age causes autism, but it could certainly be a contributing factor. Also, the National Longitudinal Survey of Youth demonstrates that television watching at three years of age and under is associated with attention problems at the age of seven, even after controlling for variables such as prenatal substance use and socioeconomic status.[52] If television may play a role in problems with attention, it is logical to question whether TV may be involved in the development of attention disorders such as attention-deficit disorder (ADD) or attention-deficit hyperactivity disorder (ADHD). Another study reveals that after adjusting for factors such as socioeconomic status and parent-child interactions, every hour spent viewing baby DVDs or videos results in infants eight to sixteen months of age acquiring six to eight fewer new words than babies who do not watch them.[53]

The bottom line is that television and DVDs/videos are over-stimulating. This is especially true for the rapidly developing minds of infants and young children. It is no wonder that children are addicted to television and video games and suffer from attention problems. They expect to be constantly entertained because, from early on, we have taught them to be highly stimulated rather than be creative or use their imaginations. Whether they are presented with toys that boast flashing lights, bells, and whistles or the constant sight and sound of the television, their senses are over-stimulated beginning soon after birth. They do not know any differently. When children are brought up accustomed to high levels of stimulation such as from the television and video games, we cannot hope that they will desire to sit down and read a book or go outside and take a walk for pleasure as they grow up and enter older childhood, adolescence, even adulthood; rather, they will demand to be entertained.

Screen Time Rules and Limits

It is apparent that children and teenagers of all ages spend much of their time in front of the television and video games. Even if they do not develop obesity during their younger years, they are establishing a dangerous habit and, in many cases, it may become an addiction. Sitting in front of a screen for hour upon hour pollutes both the mind and body. Television, movies, video games, and the Internet often contain material that is inappropriate for highly impressionable children and adolescents. Further, a sedentary lifestyle is detrimental for the body, and over time, will affect the child's health and well-being.

An acquaintance once admitted that her son is addicted to video games – to "Mario," to be exact. Unfortunately, this is not an exaggeration, nor is it rare in our society today. However, what makes the situation worse is that this boy was only three years old at the time and this woman is a health and fitness guru. This scenario illustrates that, just as it is important to develop healthy eating habits and patterns of physical activity when children are very young, parents must establish appropriate rules regarding their children's screen time exposure and use early on.

Take some time to evaluate how much television your child watches each day. How much time does he or she spend playing video games? What amount of time is spent in front of the computer, or on a smartphone? This will give you a starting point for setting screen time guidelines in your home.

Studies prove that setting screen time rules and limits works. Young children six years old and under who have rules regarding the amount of television they are allowed watch spend nearly one half-hour less watching TV each day.[54] In addition, young children whose parents always enforce their rules about screen time spend more time playing outside, are significantly more likely to read every day, and spend longer amounts of time reading. Furthermore, youth eight to eighteen years of age whose parents set media rules spend less total time exposed to media content, including TV, video games, and the computer: on average, almost three hours less per day.[55] Children who do not have a television in their bedroom, who live in a home where the TV is not on during meals or turned on when no one is watching, and whose parents set some type of rules spend considerably less time in front of a screen than kids who live in homes where media opportunities are essentially unlimited.[56]

Screen Time Recommendations

The American Academy of Pediatrics (AAP) has issued guidelines regarding screen time usage among children and adolescents. The AAP recommends that children over the age of two engage in no more than one to two hours of quality screen time per day, including TV, DVDs/videos, video games, and computer time; children under the age of two should not be exposed to any screen time at all.[57] These recommendations apply to "educational" programs and video/computer games as well. Moreover, the AAP recommends that parents remove television sets from their children's bedrooms; monitor the programs and games their children and adolescents view to ensure that they are informational, educational, and nonviolent; and watch and discuss television shows or DVDs/videos alongside their children. According to the AAP's guidelines, parents need to engage infants and toddlers in interactive activities that foster cognitive development, such as playing, reading, talking, and singing. Parents should encourage children and adolescents to participate in screen time alternatives including reading, creative play, hobbies, and sports.

Based upon the results of a survey regarding screen time and school performance, some researchers have issued stricter screen time recommendations than the AAP, and that is to limit weekday television, movie, and video game usage to one hour or less per day.[58] Additionally, the study authors strongly suggest restricting children's and adolescent's access to R-rated movies and videos as well as cable channels in order to limit exposure to adult media.

The epidemic of childhood obesity mandates that American families drastically reduce the amount of time we spend in front of the TV and other screens. A reasonable recommendation for total screen time is to limit it to less than ten hours per week. That breaks down to about one hour on weekdays and up to two hours on weekend days, which allows for movie-watching on the weekends. If your child or teenager currently spends more than ten hours per week in front of a TV, computer, video game, smartphone, and/or any other type of screen, talk about the risks of too much screen time in an age-appropriate manner, and then gradually begin to decrease screen time usage in your home.

While total screen time does not necessarily include time spent on the computer for schoolwork, when your child spends an inordinate amount of time on the computer doing homework, you might consider counting that towards part of her total screen time depending upon the amount of time, circumstances, and the particular child. Although her mind is active, she is physically inactive; her body needs to get up and move after sitting in front of the computer for a prolonged amount of time.

Babies and toddlers less than two years of age should not spend any time in front of a television or other screen, nor should they be exposed to screens, such as by simply being in a room with the TV turned on. This means that the TV should never be left on as "background noise," which has become a habit for many American families. Similarly, the radio should not regularly be on while babies and young children are playing because it is over-stimulating for them and distracts them from their play and use of language.

Many parents and caregivers often inadvertently and unknowingly encourage screen time, especially among young children, because it serves as a "babysitter." Or because they believe that the program or video/computer game is educational. However, it is ultimately a parent's responsibility to teach his or her child, not that of the TV or computer. More than that, young children learn far more by exploring, playing, being creative, using their imaginations, and looking at books than by sitting in front of a screen, no matter how educational the program or game may be. Kids learn best by interacting with their parents, caregivers, and other loved ones and by being involved in the day-to-day tasks of life – not by sitting and staring at a screen.

Television sets and all other sources of screen time need to be permanently removed from children's and adolescent's bedrooms. Furthermore, TV and other media should not be left on while eating meals or snacks, even if nobody is watching it or seems to be paying attention. The one exception to this is the occasional family movie night when everyone can enjoy eating popcorn or ice cream together while watching a movie.

As a family, agree ahead of time on the number of hours and specific programs your kids can watch, both during the week and on weekends. Let your children choose from a selection of shows or videos that you approve of. Do not allow children to watch TV just to pass the time or because they are bored. It is imperative that parents know when their children are watching television as well as what it is that they are watching. Instruct your kids to ask for permission before turning on the TV, DVDs/videos, video games, or computer; screen time should be viewed as a privilege, not a right. Allow your children to watch one or two specific programs (or play one or two specific games), and then turn off the TV or computer. As often as possible, watch what your children are viewing with them and discuss it as a family. Do not hesitate to turn off anything that seems inappropriate for your child or teenager to be viewing.

Another important habit is to analyze and critique commercials with your kids, especially those for "junk food" and fast-food. A simple way to do this is by teaching children accurate nutrition information as opposed to what may be merely "hype," misleading, or altogether false. Of course, this must be done in an age-appropriate manner, and can be particularly difficult to do with young children, but it is critical to start this practice early. Otherwise, children will often accept advertising claims as true without question. For starters, ask your child about what he or she just saw. Make kids aware that it was an advertisement intended to sell them something as a means of making money for the company, and that it might not be entirely truthful. Explain that the food in the commercial – as well as other items sold by the food manufacturer or fast-food restaurant – could be unhealthy for them. Point out that even though the commercial might be fun and entertaining to watch, or contain characters that they admire, it does not necessarily mean that the product is good for their bodies. Then discuss better, more nutritious choices.

Next, take these lessons to the grocery store and teach children to read and analyze nutrition labels for the products that they have seen advertised. Compare the actual labels to what has been viewed on television. As an example, look at the labels to determine which contains a greater amount of sugar but less fiber: original (plain) Cheerios® or Trix®? You can also evaluate fast-food versus more healthy options; for instance, do French fries or raw baby carrots have less fat and calories? The learning should continue in your own kitchen and pantry at home: It is vital to have healthy foods available at home and explain why they are better choices than those seen on TV.

These new screen time limits may very well require a new level of self-discipline among all members of your family, but that is a characteristic parents desire to instill in children and teenagers in the first place. And we cannot expect kids to develop self-control and self-discipline if we as their role models do not possess and demonstrate these behaviors ourselves. As with any behavior modification, make changes slowly and gradually; over time, they will become new habits for you and your entire family.

Screen Time Alternatives

- Be creative! Allow your kids help guide your family in making choices about alternative ways to spend your time.

- Plan a weekly family game night that does not consist of any video games. Play board games or card games; do puzzles; play Mad Libs or other interactive word games; do brain teasers or optical illusions; tell jokes to each other – use a joke book to make it more fun and interesting.

- Read together. Older children and adolescents can read aloud from a family-friendly chapter book that interests everyone. Make a trip to the library together to pick out books for this purpose.

- Make dinner together as a family. Get everyone involved in preparing the meal in some way.

- Have a picnic; if the weather does not permit an outdoor picnic, throw a blanket down on the living room floor and have a picnic there.

- Get out of the house and go watch a play, musical, ballet, or other live performance.

- Go to a concert that is age-appropriate for all family members.

- Get your child involved in an after-school activity or club.

- Visit a museum. Children's Museums, Science Centers, and History Museums are fun for kids and adults alike, plus they are engaging on both a mental and physical level.

- Go to the zoo or aquarium.

- Help your child develop talents, interests, and hobbies. Take your child to browse at a craft store if you are unsure of what might interest him. Ask your child if he would like to learn to play an instrument or take singing lessons. Photography is another idea. There is also Children's Theater, art classes, dance lessons, and on and on.

- Take a trip to the library; many libraries have structured activities for kids, such as story time.

- Check your area for local Toddler Gyms or age-appropriate gymnastics classes.

- Is your child interested in any type of sport, whether recreational, at school, or through a club or other organization?

- Get out and be active as a family. Go for a walk, hike, or bike ride; play at the park; go rollerblading or roller skating; play badminton, tennis, or basketball; go swimming; fly a kite; go play at the beach.

- Visit your local YMCA or gym, parks and recreation department, or community center. These locales usually have gyms or other open areas where kids and teenagers can run around and play, and these organizations typically offer a multitude of programs (athletic and non-athletic) for both children and adolescents.

- Refer to "Tips for Increasing Physical Activity among Children and Adolescents" at the end of the previous chapter, "Establishing Physical Activity Habits Early," for more ideas.

Too much screen time can also interfere with adequate sleep, rest, and relaxation. This is significant for multiple reasons, but as it pertains to this book, adequate sleep and rest are essential for maintaining a healthy, whole body and overall well-being. The next chapter will discuss the necessity of adequate sleep, rest, and relaxation along with ways that children and adolescents can establish healthy habits in this regard.

11 HEALTHY SLEEP, REST, & RELAXATION HABITS

Jesse, a preschooler, shifted from normal weight to overweight to obese rather quickly, despite an above average activity level. What makes the situation more puzzling is that he has no family history of weight issues, and in fact, his parents and siblings are all remarkably healthy and fit. However, there are some very interesting family dynamics involved. Jesse's siblings are considerably older than he is, so they go to bed late at night. On top of that, his parents are usually on-the-go and out past what would be an appropriate bedtime for Jesse. Further, he is involved in several extra-curricular activities, such as basketball, Tae Kwon Do, and swimming – often simultaneously – which means that he has little downtime. Making matters worse, Jesse continues to sleep in his parents' bed nearly every night, a habit that was developed early on. As a result of all of these details, this preschooler has no specific bedtime and goes to bed whenever the rest of the family does. This not only results in too little sleep, but it also causes irregular sleeping habits. The problem is that young children need significantly more sleep than older children, adolescents, and adults. This poor child tries to keep up with the rest of his family, but his body cannot meet the demands. Consequently, Jesse's body weight began to increase. And when his sleeping habits did not improve, the pounds continued to pile on.

Sleep is vital for life, a fact that is well understood. However, exactly how much sleep is necessary is less clear. Confounding the matter is that each individual requires a different amount of sleep, and not simply based on age. Some people are wired to need more sleep, while others can function well with less. Regardless, over the past few decades, the pace of life in America has become busier and more hurried; as a result, Americans – including children and adolescents – are spending less time attaining their critically needed sleep.[1,2] Interestingly, the increased rates of overweight and obesity in our nation correlate with this decline in time spent sleeping.

Fatigue and stress are detrimental to health and well-being on multiple levels; lack of rest affects physical, mental, and spiritual health. Case in point: being overly tired or stressed can contribute to unhealthy weight gain and the development of obesity. Although the causes are multi-factorial and still under investigation, hormones play a major role. For instance, individuals who do not get enough sleep produce more of the hormone ghrelin, which stimulates hunger, and less of the hormone leptin, which inhibits hunger.[3] As a result, lack of sleep leads to food cravings and an increased appetite; conversely, an adequate amount of shut-eye helps to control appetite.

However, there are additional factors involved in the relationship between sleep and weight. Those who sleep less may consume a greater amount of food and calories because they are awake for longer periods of time; they may also be more sedentary during the day due to fatigue and lack of energy.[4] Sleep-deprived individuals also tend to make poor food choices rather than eating lower-calorie, nutrient-dense foods.[5,6] Regardless of the exact cause, research proves that there is a correlation between not getting an adequate amount of sleep and the development of obesity.

Inadequate Sleep and Obesity

Sleep is crucial to well-being because it refreshes and restores the body in multiple ways. It is well-known that sleep is necessary for optimal cognitive and emotional functioning. Sleep is also essential for a healthy immune system and to ward off illness and disease.[7] Recently, several studies confirm that inadequate sleep results in adverse health outcomes, including diabetes, insulin resistance, cardiovascular disease, and a greater risk of obesity.[8] In fact, as early as infancy and toddlerhood, sleep is essential to a growing child's health and well-being.

Infants, Toddlers, and Young Children

According to Project Viva, infants and toddlers who get less than twelve hours of sleep per twenty-four hour period are twice as likely to be obese at three years of age.[9] Not surprisingly, those who watch the most television and get the least amount of sleep are at the highest risk of obesity. Another study shows that children who get the least amount of sleep each night have higher body mass indexes (BMIs) and are more likely to be overweight five years later.[10]

The Avon longitudinal study of parents and children demonstrates that when a three year old gets less than ten-and-a-half hours of sleep every night, he is more likely to be obese at the age of seven.[11] This risk is independent of other possible risk factors, such as socioeconomic status. Similarly, research reveals that children under five years old who get less than ten hours of sleep per night are almost two times more likely to be overweight or obese five years later.[12] A significant finding of this study is that sufficient sleep at night is critical; in other words, napping during the day is not an appropriate substitute for inadequate nighttime sleep in terms of obesity prevention. These results are confirmed by the Early Childhood Longitudinal Study (Birth Cohort), which found that four year olds who get at least ten-and-a-half hours of sleep each night have a lower risk of obesity.[13]

An investigation conducted among children four to ten years of age shows that those who get the least amount of sleep and/or have the most irregular sleep patterns are significantly more likely to be obese.[14] Moreover, these children exhibit metabolic abnormalities based on blood tests, including altered insulin levels. An additional discovery made by the researchers is that American children generally do not get enough sleep each night, regardless of their weight status. In children five to thirteen years of age, a lack of nighttime sleep results in a greater risk of becoming overweight, or of shifting from overweight to obese.[15]

Older Children and Adolescents

Only about one-third of adolescents meet the recommendation for nine hours of sleep per night.[16] What is more, approximately forty percent of twelve to sixteen year olds report feeling tired when they wake up.[17] Although sleep is critical during adolescence, sleep deprivation is common, largely because older children and teenagers go to bed later at night, yet get up early for school or work in the morning. In addition, the increased usage of television and movies, the computer and Internet, video games, and cellular phones/smartphones – which are often present in older children's bedrooms – all have a negative impact on their sleep habits.[18] This is true for two reasons. First, the artificial bright light emitted by the television, computers, and other technological devices interferes with the secretion of melatonin, the hormone that signals to our body that it is time to go to sleep. Second, most forms of technology are engaging and difficult to turn off. Examples include the fourteen year old who obsessively checks Facebook® to see if anyone has left a new comment regarding her most recent status update; the high school "gamer" who says he will play "just one more round" of Mortal Kombat™; and the sixteen year old who hides under the covers texting with her boyfriend long after she is supposed to be asleep. Despite the increased number of sleep-disrupting distractions, sleep is just as important for older children and adolescents as it is for infants and young children.

A National Institute of Child Health and Human Development study reveals that for every additional hour of nightly sleep a child gets in third grade, her risk of obesity in sixth grade is reduced by about forty percent, regardless of her weight status in third grade.[19] For each extra hour of sleep she gets every night in sixth grade, her chance of concurrent obesity decreases by approximately twenty percent. This remains true after adjusting for risk factors such as gender, race/ethnicity, and socioeconomic status.

Research demonstrates that obese ten to sixteen year olds sleep for a considerably shorter amount of time than their normal-weight counterparts.[20] Similarly, the Heartfelt Study found that obese eleven to sixteen year olds get less sleep than those who are not obese; that is, those with shorter sleep durations have higher BMIs and greater body fat levels.[21] For every hour of sleep that is lost in children in this age group, the risk of obesity increases by approximately eighty percent.

Among adolescents between thirteen and eighteen years of age, regularly getting at least six to eight hours of sleep at night is associated with a lower risk of obesity, even after controlling for other possible factors.[22] Adequate sleep also increases the likelihood that adolescents will engage in healthy behaviors, such as eating a nutritious diet, being physically active, and managing stress appropriately. The Cleveland Children's Sleep and Health Study found that adolescents between the ages of sixteen and nineteen who sleep less than eight hours on weeknights consume more calorie-dense snacks and high-fat foods than those who sleep longer, putting them at increased risk for becoming overweight or obese.[23] In fact, the prevalence of obesity is considerably higher among adolescents who sleep less than eight hours per weeknight.

Additional Risks of Inadequate Sleep

There are numerous negative effects of sleep deprivation, including physical, cognitive, emotional, psychological, social, and academic consequences.[24,25] As an example, several studies show that there is a correlation between lack of sleep and attention deficit/hyperactivity disorder (ADHD). Although adults usually become drowsy with too little sleep, children tend to become the opposite: hyperactive, impulsive, and aggressive.[26] Children diagnosed with ADHD may exhibit more pronounced symptoms of the disorder when they have not had enough sleep; in some cases, a child may appear to have ADHD when the issue is actually sleep deprivation.[27,28] In these instances, correcting the underlying sleep problem could theoretically reduce or eliminate hyperactivity and the associated symptoms.

Inadequate sleep can result in moodiness, irritability, anxiety, or depression among children and adolescents.[29] Lack of sleep may also lead to behavioral problems, as well as have a negative impact on school attendance.[30] Additionally, according to the American Academy of Pediatrics, sleep deprivation is associated with poor academic performance among adolescents.[31] For instance, those who earn better grades (As and Bs) report that they sleep significantly longer and have more regular sleep schedules, particularly on school nights, than those who get lower grades (Cs and below). Furthermore, older children and young adolescents who wake up tired report less motivation to do well at school; on the other hand, those who feel well-rested are highly motivated to do their best at school, have a positive image of themselves as students, and are more respectful of their teachers' influence.

Although often overlooked, driving while drowsy is a major concern for adolescents (and young adults). The number of motor vehicle accidents caused by the driver falling asleep is staggering, and studies have found that the majority of these types of accidents involve young people between the age of sixteen and twenty-nine.[32] Reports show that lack of sleep is a primary reason that individuals doze off behind the wheel. Compared to those who sleep eight or more hours per night, individuals who sleep six to seven hours a night nearly double their chances of being in a sleep-related car accident; this risk increases by four-and-a-half among those that sleep less than five hours.

Sleep Recommendations

How much sleep did your child get last night? How much sleep does he or she get on most nights of the week? You may be surprised to learn that your child is not getting nearly enough sleep. The National Sleep Foundation is an excellent resource and is available on-line at SleepFoundation.org.

According to the National Sleep Foundation, newborns (one to two months old) need a total of ten-and-a-half to eighteen hours of sleep per twenty-four hour period.[33] Infants (three to eleven months old) need nine to twelve hours of sleep each night, plus one to four thirty-minute to two hour naps during the day, for a total of about fourteen to fifteen hours every twenty-four hours. Toddlers (one to three years old) need twelve to fourteen hours of sleep in a twenty-four hour period.

Young children (three to five year olds) require eleven to thirteen hours of sleep per night, while school-aged children (five to twelve year olds) should get ten to eleven hours each night.[34] Adolescents require at least eight-and-a-half to nine-and-a-quarter hours of sleep a night;[35] possibly as much as ten, according to some researchers.[36] Adults need to aim for seven to nine hours of shut-eye per night.[37]

Encouraging Healthy Sleep Habits

As with any beneficial habit, healthy sleep habits must be taught to children and adolescents. In fact, ensuring that your child gets enough sleep may be as important to his health as a nutritious diet and regular physical activity. To help do this, make sure that your child has a quiet, dark, relaxing bedroom that is kept cool – neither too hot nor too cold.[38] Next, help your child avoid bright light in the evening, but expose him to it when he wakes in the morning. Additionally, the following steps will foster healthy sleep habits among children of all ages.

Infants (Newborn to One Year Old)[39]

- Establish a regular bedtime/naptime schedule and routine.

- Identify your infant's sleep cues, such as fussiness, crying, yawning, or rubbing her eyes. Put her down to sleep as soon as she begins to exhibit such signs.

- To help her to learn to fall asleep on her own, lay your baby down when she is drowsy, but still awake. This way, she will be more likely to go back to sleep on her own when she wakes up in the middle of the night.

- Keep her bedroom dark and quiet: avoid exposure to television and other noises.

- If your baby wakes up during the night, wait a few minutes to see if she will fall back to sleep on her own.

- To avoid arousing your baby during nighttime feedings or diaper changes, keep the room dim and refrain from over-stimulation, such as playing with her.

Toddlers and Preschoolers (One to Five Years Old)[40]

- Maintain a consistent bedtime and naptime schedule.

- A routine bedtime activity, such as taking a bath, reading a book, or saying prayers, will help your little one wind down for bed.

- Avoid letting your child nap late in the day, which may make it difficult for him to fall asleep at bedtime.

- Ensure that young children have plenty of time and space to run, jump, play, and be active; the more active kids are during the day, the better they will sleep at night (and at naptime).

- Do not allow your young one to sleep in the same bed with you because this will interfere with his ability to fall asleep on his own.

- If your child wakes up during the night, wait before responding. If he does not fall back to sleep on his own, reassure him that you are present. At the same time, do not turn on any lights or play with him. If nighttime awakenings happen frequently, gradually move farther and farther from his bed when you go to comfort him, so that eventually you can reassure him without even going into his bedroom.

School-Aged Children (Five to Twelve Years Old)[41]

- Enforce strict bedtimes and regular wake times, especially in light of the growing number commitments and activities for this age group, like school, homework, church, and sports.

- Allow your child to sleep in on the weekends, but no more than two to three hours beyond normal because this interrupts the body's internal "clock."

- Make sure your child has an appropriate, comfortable bed that is used only for sleeping. Instruct children not to use the bed for other activities, including watching television, playing video games, or eating. This trains the body that the bed is solely for rest and will aid in the process of falling asleep.

- Remove televisions, computers, video games, cellular/smart phones, and other technological devices from bedrooms. If your child or teenager requires a computer for doing homework, set it up in a location other than the bedroom.

- Encourage your child to avoid caffeinated beverages, particularly after lunch. This does not just refer to coffee; caffeine is present in a myriad of beverages popular among youth: colas and other sodas, energy drinks, tea/iced tea, and specialty beverages containing coffee, such as those from Starbucks'.

- Investigate any medications – prescription and over-the-counter – that your child takes. These may interrupt normal sleep patterns, whether by causing drowsiness during the day or insomnia at night.

- Do not allow your child to eat large meals close to bedtime. An overly-full stomach and the process of digestion can interfere with sleep.

- Ensure that your child engages in plenty of physical activity, but not within a few hours of going to bed.

- Have children avoid activities that may be physically and/or mentally stimulating near bedtime, such as intense studying, reading a thriller, exercising, playing computer games, texting, or arguing.

- Reserve the hour before bed for a quiet, relaxing activity that helps your child wind down for sleep. This includes turning off computers, phones, and other sources of technology at least one hour prior to bedtime. Reading is an appropriate nighttime activity, as long as it is not too stimulating or engrossing.

- Perhaps most important: be a good role model for your children. Establish healthy sleep habits for the whole family, and then consistently follow them.

Adolescents (Twelve to Eighteen Years Old)[42,43]

- Refer to the "School-Aged Children" section, above.

- Do not allow teenagers to stay up all night, not even to study.

- Encourage adolescents to avoid alcohol, nicotine, and other drugs, including over-the-counter and prescription medications, which can all interfere with the body's sleep-wake cycle.

If at any age your child struggles with a weight issue and also has some type of sleep problem, whether it is a difficulty with falling asleep or staying asleep – or if she consistently wakes up abnormally tired – it would be prudent to schedule an appointment with her pediatrician to determine if there is an underlying cause.

Stress and Weight

Just as with sleep deprivation, stress can lead to unhealthy weight gain for several reasons. Again, a hormone (cortisol) is a significant contributing factor. Cortisol is referred to as the "stress hormone" because the body secretes excess amounts of it during times of stress.[44,45] Cortisol seems to promote the storage of body fat, particularly around the abdomen. High levels of cortisol can also cause an increase in appetite, particularly for high-sugar foods.[46] Moreover, stressed-out individuals often make unhealthy food choices, and some turn to food for comfort – commonly referred to as emotional eating or stress eating – causing them to overeat rather than heed their hunger and fullness cues.

The best method for combating stress-related weight gain is by preventing and managing stress in the first place. Although beyond the scope of this book, effective stress prevention and management strategies are necessary to keep stress levels under control. However, one major way to prevent or manage stress is to simplify your life, to ensure that life is not overly busy or demanding and that the entire family enjoys plenty of rest and relaxation. The human body is simply not designed to go and go and go, most especially that of a growing child. Life demands balance.

Rest and Relaxation

In his book, *The Leadership Lock*, Roger Archer states that, "The demand on our life to produce, and the pressure we feel, is greater now than any time in our nation's history."[47] As a result, today's families – adults and children alike – are overworked, overstressed, and overtired. The consequences are unfathomable yet undeniable: Record numbers of children and adolescents now suffer from mood disorders, such as depression and anxiety.[48] Researchers report that this is largely due to our society's increased focus on worldly values, such as materialism and achieving a certain status, rather than core values, such as enjoying a sense of community and experiencing deep meaning in life. Essentially, children and adolescents are unable to handle the impossible demands of our fast-paced culture, which focuses almost entirely on achievement, and they are suffering beneath the weight. Parents, caregivers, and mentors must break this cycle and teach children and adolescents a different way of life – a life that includes rest, relaxation, and a break from the endless stress and pressure.

According to Roger Archer, "We have to recreate to re-create... Sometimes we must simply stop."[49] In other words, we need to rest, relax, play, have fun with our family and friends in order to refresh, revitalize, and renew our bodies and minds; this is just as true for children and adolescents as it is for adults. Be aware, though, that resting, relaxing, and having fun does not refer to being completely physically inactive day after day. Nor does it give license to sit and watch the television or play video games for hour upon hour. Quite the opposite, in fact. Use the time to take a nap, read a book, go on a leisurely walk, play board games, go to the park, have an unhurried picnic, spend time at the beach or pool, or just hang out and talk with no particular agenda.

In *What Every Child Needs,* Elisa Morgan and Carol Kuykendall recommend that parents, "Create or allow unstructured time. Don't over-schedule children in activities. Be sure they experience 'down' time to let their minds wander or to learn to enjoy their own company. Keep naptime a quiet time, even after they outgrow naps."[50] This is an ideal way to start instilling the habits of resting and relaxing in young children. Moreover, children of all ages should be allowed to just be kids with plenty of free-time and playtime; it is through play and using their imaginations that children learn and develop.

Parents demonstrate love to their children by spending quality time with them more so than by shuttling them from one activity to another. One simple step families can take to decrease the busyness in exchange for more time to rest, recuperate, and play together is to cut back on children's extracurricular activities. That means saying, "No," to some things while, at the same time, limiting other commitments. There are countless "good" opportunities and activities to be involved in, but we just cannot do them all if the goal is to be physically, emotionally, and relationally healthy and whole. The cultural mindset is that children will not develop to their fullest potential or be successful if they are not exposed to every available activity, but this is simply not true. Being involved in too many activities results in exhausted, overloaded children, adolescents, and parents; as a result, we all end up functioning poorly in other areas of life. Take time to slow down and cut out all the extra "stuff." That means enrolling children in only one activity at a time – two at the very most. This will decrease the stress in everyone's lives and give kids and families more time to rest and have fun together; it will also enable families to prepare and sit down to meals together on a regular basis, as discussed in chapter seven, "More Family Meals, Less Happy Meals®."

The Role of Technology

In the quest to simplify day-to-day life, our lives have become increasingly complicated. Advances in technology have negated any opportunity for families to truly rest, relax, and recreate. Think about the realities of life today. It is nearly impossible to completely disconnect from work these days, even when at home in the evening or over the weekend. In the same way, families cannot really get away on vacation anymore. In the long-run, technology actually adds to the busyness and stress of life, rather than making it easier as originally intended. Because we can supposedly do more in less time, and do it from anywhere, we place more on an already overflowing plate – often without hesitation. And because technology is moving at a rate faster than ever before, these issues are only going to become more pronounced.

Besides being a major cause of car accidents, cellular phones require us to be available to everyone, including employers, twenty-four hours a day, seven days per week. E-mail serves the same purpose. Call-waiting enables us to talk to two people at once. Whose life are we making easier – ours or the individual who is trying to get ahold of us? It is not beneficial to one's mental health to virtually be available to the whole world one hundred percent of the time.

Computers help us work faster, causing us to take on more work. Laptops and tablets allow us to work while out of the office or away from home, even while "on vacation." The Internet enables us to research anything at any time – day or night – from the comfort of our own home; wireless Internet enables us to do it at Starbucks®, where we would prefer to relax over a cup of coffee with a friend. Smart phones merely magnify the problem. The list goes on and on.

As mentioned in chapter nine, "Establishing Physical Activity Habits Early," most of the modern-day conveniences meant to save time result in less physical exertion. Activities that would normally expend calories no longer do. Although it may only be a few calories here and there, the calorie disparity adds up over time: twisting a manual can opener, taking the stairs instead of the elevator, getting up and walking across the room instead of using a remote control, walking or biking instead of driving. As a result, we need to spend an hour at the gym to stay physically fit. In the end, little time is saved.

Modern technology need not be abandoned; I use it on a daily basis and am very grateful for the convenience. However, Americans need to be aware of these issues and how technology affects our lives in numerous ways, not all of them positive. Rest, relaxation, and peace of mind will not come until we slow down, take breaks, and make time to have fun with our families.

The bottom line is that obtaining an adequate amount of sleep, rest, and relaxation is an effective remedy for numerous problems that the human body may suffer from, including overweight, obesity, and many illnesses. Regardless, today's cultural norms make getting an appropriate amount of sleep and rest difficult to do, and it will require dramatic changes in many American homes to reverse this trend. As a matter of fact, the following chapter addresses several lifestyle practices that underlie the obesity epidemic; these behaviors and attitudes have subtly become customary because of a shift in modern-day cultural values.

12 A BYPRODUCT OF OUR CULTURE

Obesity is not only becoming more prevalent in the United States – it is growing more common among many other developed and developing nations as well.[1,2] In fact, it is reaching epidemic levels worldwide.[3] The most recent estimates by the World Health Organization reveal that one-and-a-half billion adults around the world are overweight; this includes approximately five hundred million that are classified as obese, which means that over ten percent of the world's adult population is *obese*.[4] Furthermore, obesity among preschoolers, school-aged children, and adolescents has become a grave concern internationally.[5,6] The International Obesity Taskforce estimates that, globally, approximately one in ten school-aged children – as many as two hundred million – are overweight or obese.[7,8] This figure is equivalent to the total number of children living in the United States multiplied by two-and-a-half. What is more, forty to fifty million of these youngsters are obese – more than the entire population of Canada.[9] It is also estimated that, worldwide, close to forty-three million children under the age of five are affected by this growing problem.[10]

The widespread epidemic of overweight and obesity is a byproduct of American culture: As other countries become industrialized and "Westernized" – more like the United States – their citizens begin to experience a greater prevalence of obesity and weight-related health problems.[11] The adoption of a "Western" lifestyle includes increased consumption of high-calorie convenience and fast-foods, as well as a less active lifestyle. For example, although fast-food chains originated in the United States, McDonald's® has expanded to more than thirty-one thousand restaurants in over one hundred and nineteen countries (more than half of the countries in the world);[12] Burger King® has over eleven thousand locations in sixty-one countries (nearly one-third of the countries in the world).[13]

One striking example of the influence our nation has had on other countries is in China, where an obesity epidemic has developed among all population and age groups.[14] This has occurred relatively recently and over a brief period of time.[15,16] The Chinese used to be some of the most fit and healthy individuals in the world, but they are quickly becoming like those who reside in America.[17] As a result, China now has a higher incidence of obesity-related diseases than ever before, including type 2 diabetes, cardiovascular disease, high blood pressure, and stroke.[18,19] Even worse, a national public health problem has developed because of the serious medical and psychological consequences that obese Chinese children are suffering from.[20]

The new issues China is experiencing have been blamed on lifestyle changes among the Chinese, namely those related to diet and physical activity.[21,22] They have made changes to their traditional diet, including a higher intake of fat; decreased their amount of daily physical activity, such as a greater reliance on motorized transportation; and adopted a sedentary way of life, including less active jobs and increased computer, television, and video game usage.[23,24] Essentially, the lifestyle of the Chinese has become increasingly similar to that of Americans – to the detriment of their health. This puts America to shame.

As they become more Westernized, otherwise healthy cultures are beginning to experience weight and health problems identical to those in the United States. It is painfully clear that *our* culture is to blame as the cause of this worldwide epidemic. As will be explained shortly, the issues of childhood and adult obesity and chronic disease are nothing more than a symptom of the fragmented culture in America.

Poison can be insidious, undetected; but it is deadly all the same. Similarly, behaviors and attitudes that subtly become accepted and pervasive in a subculture can, at times, be harmful to its members' health and well-being. Examples of this can be seen in history and present-day, both in American society as well as other cultures. Extreme illustrations include college rush week hosted by fraternal organizations, hazing as a rite of initiation into a group, scarification and other body-altering practices, and strict devotees of the raw foods movement. To outsiders, the beliefs and behaviors of these specific groups are risky, bizarre, even abhorrent. But to those that belong, their activities have evolved into a normal way of life. Albeit a stretch, there is a parallel between this and the eating and physical activity habits of Americans. What has become acceptable in American society is actually detrimental to our health and well-being. To someone from another culture, the lifestyle habits we have developed are shocking, inexplicable, harmful. In contrast, consider the Amish. It is rare to see an obese Amish person because they have not succumbed to modern-day culture or its inherent byproducts. At the very least, this is a thought-provoking truth.

The Root Causes of Childhood Obesity

In every area of life, there are direct and indirect repercussions for our actions. We demonstrate this to our children when we reward them for desirable behavior and discipline them when they misbehave. It is extremely clear that our country has become derailed, in a number of ways, from the track towards good health and overall well-being. Because we have gotten off of this path and tried to make our own way, society is reaping the consequences: an epidemic of overweight and obesity along with the related health problems. Before we can begin to wage battle against childhood obesity, we need to examine ourselves and determine whether or not we are ready to make significant changes in order to get back on track. Otherwise, our nation – especially our children and our children's children – will pay severely, both directly and indirectly.

The ten topics discussed in the preceding chapters are the result of various attitudes and behaviors prevalent in current American society. These underlying issues indirectly – yet largely – contribute to the epidemic of childhood obesity. Examples of these root causes are materialism, decreased emphasis on family and family values, busyness, a dependence upon technology and screens, and an unhealthy obsession with food *and* thinness.

Materialism

To begin with, America has become an overly materialistic society; our desire to accumulate wealth and possessions has surpassed our desire to raise strong, healthy families. As Roger Archer asks in his book, "Where do you spend your time and where do you spend your money? It will show you what you love."[25] In a sense, our actions convey that making money and acquiring "things" are more important than family. But it has not necessarily been a conscious decision. Cultural values have led Americans to believe that we *need* the nice things that, realistically, we do not really need. Rather, we simply *want* them: We want bigger, better, nicer, and more. And because we live in America, we know we can get these things if we work hard enough. Anything and everything is accessible to us if we are willing to pay the price. Unfortunately, many are willing to pay the price.

The materialistic mindset of our nation is indirectly breeding a generation of unhealthy and overweight children, and if we do not make adjustments, it will only grow worse. This necessitates that Americans begin living modestly, within our means; a simple lifestyle needs to become the standard. Our family's health and well-being are more important than our income, the house in which we live, or the car that we drive. When Americans stop striving to make more money in pursuit of "things," mothers and fathers will be able to spend more time at home with their families. This will not only improve the physical health of our families, but it will result in better emotional, mental, social, behavioral, and spiritual health as well.

Decreased Emphasis on Family and Family Values

Family and family values have become less of a priority in America, as illustrated by the increasing numbers of mothers working outside of the home full-time or more, along with the growing proportion of fathers working more than the normal forty hours per week. This is largely a result of our materialistic nature and desire to accumulate possessions; it is a means of earning more money to pay for nicer "things." Again, look at your calendar and your pocketbook: Where you spend your time and money is indicative of what is most valuable to you.

Because family is no longer a top priority, unhealthy habits have become commonplace in American homes. It is next to impossible for working moms to plan, shop for, and prepare healthy breakfasts, lunches, snacks, and family dinners. In turn, families have come to rely on unwholesome convenience foods and eating out, as well as items sold at school or daycare. An additional outcome is that mothers lack the time and energy to breastfeed their babies, not to mention to prepare wholesome baby and toddler foods. As a result of fathers working too many hours, kids are growing up without a father present to set a healthy example, and mothers lack the help and support they need to ensure that the family is served nutritious meals. Furthermore, ensuring that the entire family maintains beneficial lifestyle habits, like engaging in regular physical activity, limiting screen time, and getting adequate sleep, rest, and relaxation, are some of the least concerns among moms and dads who work inordinate numbers of hours.

If the epidemic of childhood obesity is not sufficient to convince Americans that we need to transform our ways, *Working Mother* magazine has published research revealing that a growing number of working mothers are abusing alcohol – including wine, or prescription drugs – such as Xanax, in order to cope with the stresses they face at work and home. Further, these moms are successful in hiding their addiction from family, friends, and coworkers. According to the survey, forty percent of working moms report that they consume alcohol, while fifty-seven percent admit to misusing prescription medications as a means of trying to deal with the pressure in their lives.[26]

Statistics cited by the article show that the number of women (between thirty and forty-four) who abuse alcohol has doubled in the last decade, while the abuse of prescription medications has increased by four hundred percent over the same time period.[27] Additionally, one in four children has a parent who is addicted to alcohol.

It is painfully evident that working mothers are overscheduled, overworked, and overstressed. This is oftentimes the case for stay-at-home moms, never mind those who work outside of the home. As an increasing number of moms take on the role of primary provider, the pressure is amplified. Many women are simply trying to do too much, and in the end, when they cannot handle it, they may turn to alcohol or prescription drugs to try and cope. This is yet another by-product of our culture that clearly demonstrates the need for change.

Being Overly Busy

It is no secret that Americans lead extremely fast-paced lives. This issue is discussed in elsewhere in this book, so it will not be expanded upon here. However, it should be noted that being overly busy contributes to the growing rate of obesity in a number of ways. Particularly, busyness results in a lack of time to: plan and prepare healthy breakfasts, lunches, and snacks; cook and sit down to well-balanced family dinners; be physically active; and get adequate sleep, rest, and relaxation. High stress levels, which also contribute to obesity, are another direct result of overscheduled, quick-paced lifestyles. The current state of our children's health requires that we slow down – that we simplify our lives – by decreasing the number of activities that our kids are involved in, as well as by limiting our own commitments outside of the home.

Dependence upon Technology and Screens

Nowadays, life revolves around technology and the accompanying screens. Americans of all ages are surrounded and inundated by electronic devices – and are becoming increasingly addicted to them. These forms of technology have, in a sense, taken over our lives and we have become dependent upon them. It is now virtually impossible to entirely detach from work, communication, the demands of others, and stress. An over-usage of technology and screens contributes to obesity in at least two ways: it leads to decreased amounts of physical activity and it interferes with the ability to rest and relax. In addition, "screen time" can make it difficult to obtain adequate amounts of sleep, especially for youth. Television, in particular, has further indirect links to the obesity epidemic, as discussed in chapter ten, "Too Much Screen Time." Parents must make a deliberate decision that our families will spend less time in front of these electronic screens and more time out being active and having fun. There is no alternative.

Obsession with Food and Thinness

Americans have been programmed to focus on food, which has turned food into an idol in our lives. We either love food – leading to gluttony and overeating, or fear food – leading to fad diets, unhealthy weight control practices, and the categorization of foods as "good" or "bad." These attitudes and actions cause us to be enslaved to food: In a sense, we put food on a pedestal and worship it. When we regularly indulge, constantly think about food, or overeat, we love and adore food. Conversely, by religiously avoiding certain foods because they are "too fattening" or "too high in calories," we fear and demonize food. These mindsets give power to the food itself and allow food to control us.

At the same time, our culture worships thinness. We watch *America's Next Top Model* and compare ourselves to the impossible-to-attain images on the screen while eating from a bucket of fried chicken that sits atop our lap. We are also captivated – rather than appalled – by the advertisements for greasy burgers and onion rings, interspersed with those for weight-loss drinks, throughout the show. There is no question as to why eating disorders and other unsafe weight loss methods are on the rise in our country. Rather than placing a focus on food, fad diets, or being "thin," we must emphasize the importance of living healthy, well-balanced lives – and help our children to do the same.

Drastic Times Call for Drastic Measures

Doctor Paul Reisser's answer to a reader's question in *Focus on the Family Magazine* summarizes several main points of this book. The question is: "What do you see as the biggest obstacle to a healthy lifestyle?" Doctor Reisser replies, "Do you have too little time to get eight hours of sleep, a half-hour of exercise, a half-hour of quiet time, and at least one unhurried meal to share with your family or friends every day? If so, your greatest obstacle to good health may not be a family history of heart disease or cancer or a love of fatty food, but rather your calendar."[28] He continues, "Wall-to-wall commitments, a frantic lifestyle, two or three jobs (or one job with the demands of two or three), constant noise, too much stuff, mounting debt, nonstop messages flooding your mental inbox, and a constant state of fatigue and anxiety – these are manifestations of living without margin." Doctor Reisser goes on to explain that living without margin is defined by author Doctor Richard Swenson as the space between: "our load and our limits," "breathing freely and suffocating," and "rest and exhaustion."

Doctor Reisser concludes his answer by asking, "Can you guess what usually gets shoved aside when the schedule is jammed?" He answers: "Not only sleep, exercise, and good nutrition, but also the time we need to nurture relationships with spouse, children, friends, and God. Bottom line: Creating margin in your life may be your most important health project."[29]

As discussed in chapter two, "Family and Parental Responsibility," parents must make children a primary concern, place them at the top of our priority list, and be present for them. This requires making time for our kids, which entails lightening every family member's overloaded schedule in an effort to create a less hectic lifestyle. This, in turn, will create "margin" in our lives, which is the first step in fighting the battle against the epidemic of obesity. As a result, parents will have the time, energy, and innate desire to establish healthy lifestyle habits that will prevent or reverse obesity among their family members. When this happens, the behaviors necessary to wage the war will materialize in our daily lives. Our arsenals will become full of positive habits such as breastfeeding and making wholesome homemade foods for babies and toddlers; teaching children to eat healthfully from the very beginning of their lives; planning and preparing nutritious breakfasts, lunches, snacks, and dinners; eating out less frequently; cooking and sitting down for healthy meals together as a family; instilling a routine of being physically active starting during children's early years; decreasing "screen time" in our homes; slowing down our pace of life and obtaining sufficient amounts of sleep, rest, and relaxation. Because of the mindsets and attitudes that have become widely accepted as normal in modern culture, these behavior changes may seem drastic, but in reality, they are not. They strengthen the body, mind, and spirit – and the rewards gained from putting them into practice are innumerable. Nonetheless, "drastic times call for drastic measures."

The epidemic of childhood obesity qualifies as a "drastic time," thus we need to pursue "drastic measures." The health of our children – the health of our nation – depends upon it. For those who are concerned about well-being of our children, our children's children, and future generations – for those who desire to leave a lasting legacy of vibrant life and good health – it will require taking a stand against what has unwittingly become today's cultural norms. The good news is that Americans are more aware of this problem than ever before, which means that more steps can and will be taken to prevent and reverse the epidemic of childhood obesity. If every individual fulfills his or her responsibility, the tide will turn and generations of youngsters will be enabled to enjoy lives full of health and wellness. Let us begin fighting the battle today.

REFERENCES

PREFACE

1 "Diet." *American Heritage Dictionary of the English Language*. Houghton Mifflin. Available at: http://education.yahoo.com/reference/dictionary/entry/diet. Accessed August 29, 2010.

2 "Diet." *American Heritage Dictionary of the English Language*. Houghton Mifflin. Available at: http://education.yahoo.com/reference/dictionary/entry/diet. Accessed August 29, 2010.

3 "Diet." *Encarta Thesaurus [English Edition]*. Microsoft. Available at: http://encarta.msn.com/encnet/features/dictionary/DictionaryResults.aspx?lextype=2&search=diet. Accessed August 29, 2010.

4 "Nutrition." *American Heritage Dictionary of the English Language*. Houghton Mifflin. Available at: http://education.yahoo.com/reference/dictionary/entry/nutrition. Accessed September 10, 2010.

5 "Nutrition." *Encarta Thesaurus [English Edition]*. Microsoft. Available at: http://encarta.msn.com/encnet/features/dictionary/DictionaryResults.aspx?lextype=2&search=nutrition. Accessed September 10, 2010.

CHAPTER 1: THE POISONING OF OUR CHILDREN

1 Reilly JJ, Armstrong J, Dorosty AR, Emmett PM, Ness A, Rogers I, Steer C, Sherriff A. Early life risk factors for obesity in childhood: Cohort study. *BMJ*. 2005;330:1357-1359.

2 Daniels SR, Arnett DK, Eckel RH, Gidding SS, Hayman LL, Kumanyika S, Robinson TN, Scott BJ, St. Jeor S, Williams CL. Overweight in children and adolescents: Pathophysiology, consequences, prevention, and treatment. *Circulation*. 2005;111:1999-2012.

3 Wang Y, Lobstein T. Worldwide trends in childhood overweight and obesity. *International Journal of Pediatric Obesity*. 2006;1:11-25.

4 Daniels SR, Arnett DK, Eckel RH, Gidding SS, Hayman LL, Kumanyika S, Robinson TN, Scott BJ, St. Jeor S, Williams CL. Overweight in children and adolescents: Pathophysiology, consequences, prevention, and treatment. *Circulation*. 2005;111:1999-2012.

5 Wang Y, Lobstein T. Worldwide trends in childhood overweight and obesity. *International Journal of Pediatric Obesity*. 2006;1:11-25.

6 Krebs NF, Himes JH, Jacobson D, Nicklas TA, Guilday P, Styne D. Assessment of child and adolescent overweight and obesity. *Pediatrics*. 2007;120:S193-S228.

7 Krebs NF, Himes JH, Jacobson D, Nicklas TA, Guilday P, Styne D. Assessment of child and adolescent overweight and obesity. *Pediatrics*. 2007;120:S193-S228.

8 National Institutes of Health (NIH), National Heart, Lung, and Blood Institute (NHLBI), NHLBI Obesity Education Initiative, North American Association for the Study of Obesity. *The Practical Guide: Identification, Evaluation, and Treatment of Overweight and Obesity in Adults*. Bethseda, MD: NIH; 2000:1,10.

9 Pi-Sunyer FX, Editor. *Clinical Management of Obesity: With Special Attention to Type 2 Diabetes*. Alexandria, VA: American Diabetes Association; 2004:9.

10 National Center for Health Statistics, National Center for Chronic Disease Prevention and Health Promotion, Centers for Disease Control and Prevention. *Clinical Growth Charts, Set 1: Children 2-20 years (5th-95th percentile), Boys BMI-for-age*. Available at: http://www.cdc.gov/growthcharts/clinical_charts.htm#Set1. Accessed September 4, 2010. Reprinted by Permission of the Centers for Disease Control and Prevention.

11 Krebs NF, Himes JH, Jacobson D, Nicklas TA, Guilday P, Styne D. Assessment of child and adolescent overweight and obesity. *Pediatrics*. 2007;120:S193-S228.

12 Olshansky SJ, Passaro DJ, Hershow RC, Layden J, Carnes BA, Brody J, Hayflick L, RN Butler, Allison DB, Ludwig DS. A potential decline in life expectancy in the United States in the 21st century. *New Engl J Med*. 2005;352:1138-1145.

13 Malik VS, Schulze MB, Hu FB. Intake of sugar-sweetened beverages and weight gain: A systematic review. *Am J Clin Nutr*. 2006;84:274-288.

14 United States Department of Health and Human Services. *The Surgeon General's Call to Action to Prevent and Decrease Overweight and Obesity*. Rockville, MD: United States Department of Health and Human Services, Public Health Service, Office of the Surgeon General; 2001.

15 Daniels SR, Arnett DK, Eckel RH, Gidding SS, Hayman LL, Kumanyika S, Robinson TN, Scott BJ, St. Jeor S, Williams CL. Overweight in children and adolescents: Pathophysiology, consequences, prevention, and treatment. *Circulation*. 2005;111:1999-2012.

16 Ogden CL, Carroll MD. National Center for Health Statistics, Centers for Disease Control and Prevention, Health E-Stats. *Prevalence of overweight, obesity and extreme obesity among adults: United States, trends 1960-62 through 2007-2008*. Available at: http://www.cdc.gov/nchs/data/hestat/obesity_adult_07_08/obesity_adult_07_08.htm. Accessed January 17, 2012.

17 Ogden CL, Carroll MD. National Center for Health Statistics, Centers for Disease Control and Prevention, Health E-Stats. *Prevalence of overweight, obesity and extreme obesity among adults: United States, trends 1960-62 through 2007-2008*. Available at: http://www.cdc.gov/nchs/data/hestat/obesity_adult_07_08/obesity_adult_07_08.htm. Accessed January 17, 2012.

18 American Academy of Pediatrics, Committee on School Health. Policy Statement: Soft drinks in schools. *Pediatrics*. 2004;113:152-154.

19 Janssen I, Katzmarzyk PT, Boyce WF, Vereecken C, Mulvihill, Roberts C, Currie C, Pickett W, The Health Behaviour in School-Aged Children Obesity Working Group. Comparison of overweight and obesity prevalence in school-aged youth from 34 countries and their relationships with physical activity and dietary patterns. *Obesity Reviews*. 2005;6:123-132.

20 Ogden C, Carroll M. National Center for Health Statistics, Centers for Disease Control and Prevention, Health E-Stats. *Prevalence of obesity among children and adolescents: United States, trends 1963-1965 through 2007-2008*. Available at: http://www.cdc.gov/nchs/data/hestat/obesity_child_07_08/obesity_child_07_08.htm. Accessed September 3, 2010.

21 Ogden C, Carroll M. National Center for Health Statistics, Centers for Disease Control and Prevention, Health E-Stats. *Prevalence of obesity among children and adolescents: United States, trends 1963-1965 through 2007-2008*. Available at: http://www.cdc.gov/nchs/data/hestat/obesity_child_07_08/obesity_child_07_08.htm. Accessed September 3, 2010.

22 Ogden C, Carroll M. National Center for Health Statistics, Centers for Disease Control and Prevention, Health E-Stats. *Prevalence of obesity among children and adolescents: United States, trends 1963-1965 through 2007-2008*. Available at: http://www.cdc.gov/nchs/data/hestat/obesity_child_07_08/obesity_child_07_08.htm. Accessed September 3, 2010. Reprinted by Permission of the Centers for Disease Control and Prevention.

23 National Institutes of Health (NIH), National Heart, Lung, and Blood Institute (NHLBI), NHLBI Obesity Education Initiative, North American Association for the Study of Obesity. *The Practical Guide: Identification, Evaluation, and Treatment of Overweight and Obesity in Adults.* Bethseda, MD: NIH; 2000:5.

24 Olshansky SJ, Passaro DJ, Hershow RC, Layden J, Carnes BA, Brody J, Hayflick L, RN Butler, Allison DB, Ludwig DS. A potential decline in life expectancy in the United States in the 21st century. *New Engl J Med.* 2005;352:1138-1145.

25 Daniels SR, Arnett DK, Eckel RH, Gidding SS, Hayman LL, Kumanyika S, Robinson TN, Scott BJ, St. Jeor S, Williams CL. Overweight in children and adolescents: Pathophysiology, consequences, prevention, and treatment. *Circulation.* 2005;111:1999-2012.

26 National Institutes of Health (NIH), National Heart, Lung, and Blood Institute (NHLBI), NHLBI Obesity Education Initiative, North American Association for the Study of Obesity. *The Practical Guide: Identification, Evaluation, and Treatment of Overweight and Obesity in Adults.* Bethseda, MD: NIH; 2000:5.

27 Flegal KM, Graubard BI, Williamson DF, Gail MH. Cause-specific excess deaths associated with underweight, overweight, and obesity. *JAMA.* 2007; 298:2028-2037.

28 Flegal KM, Graubard BI, Williamson DF, Gail MH. Cause-specific excess deaths associated with underweight, overweight, and obesity. *JAMA.* 2007; 298:2028-2037.

29 National Institutes of Health (NIH), National Heart, Lung, and Blood Institute (NHLBI), NHLBI Obesity Education Initiative, North American Association for the Study of Obesity. *The Practical Guide: Identification, Evaluation, and Treatment of Overweight and Obesity in Adults.* Bethseda, MD: NIH; 2000:5.

30 United States Department of Health and Human Services. *The Surgeon General's Call to Action to Prevent and Decrease Overweight and Obesity.* Rockville, MD: United States Department of Health and Human Services, Public Health Service, Office of the Surgeon General; 2001:8-9.

31 United States Department of Health and Human Services. *The Surgeon General's Call to Action to Prevent and Decrease Overweight and Obesity.* Rockville, MD: United States Department of Health and Human Services, Public Health Service, Office of the Surgeon General; 2001:8-9.

32 Ebbeling CB, Pawlak DB, Ludwig DS. Childhood obesity: public-health crisis, common sense cure. *Lancet.* 2002;360:473-482.

33 American Academy of Pediatrics, Committee on Nutrition. Policy Statement: Prevention of pediatric overweight and obesity. *Pediatrics.* 2003;112;424-430.

34 Rampersaud GC, Pereira MA, Girard BL, Adams J, Metzl JD. Breakfast habits, nutritional status, body weight, and academic performance in children and adolescents. *J Am Diet Assoc.* 2005;105:743-760.

35 Rampersaud GC, Pereira MA, Girard BL, Adams J, Metzl JD. Breakfast habits, nutritional status, body weight, and academic performance in children and adolescents. *J Am Diet Assoc.* 2005;105:743-760.

36 Wang Y, Lobstein T. Worldwide trends in childhood overweight and obesity. *International Journal of Pediatric Obesity.* 2006;1:11-25.

37 Krebs NF, Himes JH, Jacobson D, Nicklas TA, Guilday P, Styne D. Assessment of child and adolescent overweight and obesity. *Pediatrics.* 2007;120:S193-S228.

38 Spruyt K, Molfese DL, Gozal D. Sleep duration, sleep regularity, body weight, and metabolic homeostasis in school-aged children. Pediatrics. 2011;127:e345-e352.

39 American Academy of Pediatrics, Committee on Nutrition. Policy Statement: Prevention of pediatric overweight and obesity. *Pediatrics.* 2003;112;424-430.

40 Krebs NF, Himes JH, Jacobson D, Nicklas TA, Guilday P, Styne D. Assessment of child and adolescent overweight and obesity. *Pediatrics.* 2007;120:S193-S228.

41 Ebbeling CB, Pawlak DB, Ludwig DS. Childhood obesity: Public-health crisis, common sense cure. *Lancet.* 2002;360:473-482.

42 Krebs NF, Himes JH, Jacobson D, Nicklas TA, Guilday P, Styne D. Assessment of child and adolescent overweight and obesity. *Pediatrics.* 2007;120:S193-S228.

43 Olshansky SJ, Passaro DJ, Hershow RC, Layden J, Carnes BA, Brody J, Hayflick L, RN Butler, Allison DB, Ludwig DS. A potential decline in life expectancy in the United States in the 21st century. *New Engl J Med.* 2005;352:1138-1145.

44 United States Department of Health and Human Services. *The Surgeon General's Call to Action to Prevent and Decrease Overweight and Obesity.* Rockville, MD: United States Department of Health and Human Services, Public Health Service, Office of the Surgeon General; 2001:1.

45 American Academy of Pediatrics, Committee on Nutrition. Policy Statement: Prevention of pediatric overweight and obesity. *Pediatrics.* 2003;112:424-430.

46 Pi-Sunyer FX, Editor. *Clinical Management of Obesity: With Special Attention to Type 2 Diabetes.* Alexandria, VA: American Diabetes Association; 2004:5.

47 Taveras EM, Rifas-Shiman SL, Berkey CS, Rocket HR, Field AE, Frazier AL, Colditz GA, Gillman MW. Family dinner and adolescent overweight. *Obes Res.* 2005;13:900–906.

48 United States Department of Health and Human Services. *The Surgeon General's Call to Action to Prevent and Decrease Overweight and Obesity.* Rockville, MD: United States Department of Health and Human Services, Public Health Service, Office of the Surgeon General; 2001:1.

49 Krebs NF, Himes JH, Jacobson D, Nicklas TA, Guilday P, Styne D. Assessment of child and adolescent overweight and obesity. *Pediatrics.* 2007;120:S193-S228.

50 United States Department of Health and Human Services. *The Surgeon General's Call to Action to Prevent and Decrease Overweight and Obesity.* Rockville, MD: United States Department of Health and Human Services, Public Health Service, Office of the Surgeon General; 2001:1.

51 Pi-Sunyer FX, Editor. *Clinical Management of Obesity: With Special Attention to Type 2 Diabetes.* Alexandria, VA: American Diabetes Association; 2004:5.

52 Pi-Sunyer FX, Editor. *Clinical Management of Obesity: With Special Attention to Type 2 Diabetes.* Alexandria, VA: American Diabetes Association; 2004:7,9.

CHAPTER 2: FAMILY & PARENTAL RESPONSIBLITY

1 Frezon P. Breakfast of champions. *Guideposts Magazine.* October 2010; 65:76-80. Reprinted by permission of *Guideposts M agazine.*

2 Daniels SR, Arnett DK, Eckel RH, Gidding SS, Hayman LL, Kumanyika S, Robinson TN, Scott BJ, St. Jeor S, Williams CL. Overweight in children and adolescents: Pathophysiology, consequences, prevention, and treatment. *Circulation.* 2005;111:1999-2012.

3 Olshansky SJ, Passaro DJ, Hershow RC, Layden J, Carnes BA, Brody J, Hayflick L, RN Butler, Allison DB, Ludwig DS. A potential decline in life expectancy in the United States in the 21st century. *New Engl J Med.* 2005;352:1138-1145.

4 Peters R. *It's Never Too Soon to Discipline: A Low-Stress Program That Shows Parents How to Teach Good Behavior That Will Last a Lifetime.* New York, NY: St. Martin's Press; 1998:24.

5 Peters R. *It's Never Too Soon to Discipline: A Low-Stress Program That Shows Parents How to Teach Good Behavior That Will Last a Lifetime.* New York, NY: St. Martin's Press; 1998:47.

6 Fields LL. Five myths of parenting – parent traps. *ParentLife.* April 2010;16:30. Reprinted by Permission of WaterBrook Press.

7 Peters R. *It's Never Too Soon to Discipline: A Low-Stress Program That Shows Parents How to Teach Good Behavior That Will Last a Lifetime.* New York, NY: St. Martin's Press; 1998:71-72.

8 "Self-control." *American Heritage Dictionary of the English Language.* Houghton Mifflin. Available at: http://education.yahoo.com/reference/dictionary/entry/self-control. Accessed September 23, 2010.

9 "Self-control." *Encarta Thesaurus [English Edition].* Microsoft. Available at: http://encarta.msn.com/encnet/features/dictionary/DictionaryResults.aspx?lextype=2&search=self%2dcontrol. Accessed September 23, 2010.

10 Peters R. *It's Never Too Soon to Discipline: A Low-Stress Program That Shows Parents How to Teach Good Behavior That Will Last a Lifetime.* New York, NY: St. Martin's Press; 1998:39-40.

11 Peters R. *It's Never Too Soon to Discipline: A Low-Stress Program That Shows Parents How to Teach Good Behavior That Will Last a Lifetime.* New York, NY: St. Martin's Press; 1998:45.

12 Dobson J. *The New Dare to Discipline.* Wheaton, IL: Tyndale House Publishers, Inc.; 1992:6. Reprinted by Permission of Tyndale House Publishers.

13 Dobson J. *The New Dare to Discipline.* Wheaton, IL: Tyndale House Publishers, Inc.; 1992:14-15. Reprinted by Permission of Tyndale House Publishers.

14 Morgan E, Kuykendall C. *What Every Mom Needs.* Grand Rapids, MI: Zondervan; 1995:135-136. Reprinted by Permission of MOPS International.

15 Reilly JJ, Armstrong J, Dorosty AR, Emmett PM, Ness A, Rogers I, Steer C, Sherriff A. Early life risk factors for obesity in childhood: Cohort study. *BMJ.* 2005;330:1357-1359.

16 Krebs NF, Himes JH, Jacobson D, Nicklas TA, Guilday P, Styne D. Assessment of child and adolescent overweight and obesity. *Pediatrics.* 2007;120:S193-228.

17 Whitaker RC, Wright JA, Pepe MS, Seidel KD, Dietz WH. Predicting obesity in young adulthood from childhood and parental obesity. *N Engl J Med.* 1997;337:869-873.

18 Morgan E, Kuykendall C. *What Every Child Needs: Meet Your Child's Nine Basic Needs for Love.* Grand Rapids, MI: Zondervan; 1997:70. Reprinted by Permission of MOPS International.

19 Edelman MW. *The Measure of Our Success.* Boston, MA: Beacon Press; 1992:75. Reprinted by Permission of Beacon Press, Boston.

20 "Train." *Encarta Thesaurus [English Edition].* Microsoft. Available at: http://encarta.msn.com/thesaurus_561591357/train.html. Accessed September 30, 2010.

21 American Academy of Pediatrics, Committee on Nutrition. Policy Statement: Prevention of pediatric overweight and obesity. *Pediatrics.* 2003;112;424-430.

22 Larson NI, Story M, Eisenberg ME, Neumark-Sztainer D. Food preparation and purchasing roles among adolescents: associations with sociodemographic characteristics and diet quality. *J Am Diet Assoc.* 2006;106:211-218.

CHAPTER 3: BREASTFEEDING IS THE BEST START

1 Meek JY, Editor. *American Academy of Pediatrics New Mother's Guide to Breastfeeding.* New York, NY: Bantam Books; 2002:Dedication Page.

2 Meek JY, Editor. *American Academy of Pediatrics New Mother's Guide to Breastfeeding.* New York, NY: Bantam Books; 2002:3.

3 Meek JY, Editor. *American Academy of Pediatrics New Mother's Guide to Breastfeeding.* New York, NY: Bantam Books; 2002:3.

4 Meek JY, Editor. *American Academy of Pediatrics New Mother's Guide to Breastfeeding.* New York, NY: Bantam Books; 2002:3.

5 La Leche League International. *The Womanly Art of Breastfeeding. Seventh Revised Edition.* Schaumburg, IL: La Leche League International; 2003:6,379.

6 Wolf JH. Low breastfeeding rates and public health in the United States. *Am J Public Health.* 2003;93:2000-2008.

7 United States Department of Health and Human Services, Office on Women's Health. *National Breastfeeding Campaign Ad Council Materials.* Available at: http://www.womenshealth.gov/breast-feeding/government-programs/national-breastfeeding-campaign/adcouncil/ Accessed October 26, 2010. Reprinted by Permission of the Office on Women's Health.

8 United States Department of Health and Human Services, Office on Women's Health. *National Breastfeeding Campaign Ad Council Materials.* Available at: http://www.womenshealth.gov/breast-feeding/government-programs/national-breastfeeding-campaign/adcouncil/ Accessed October 26, 2010. Reprinted by Permission of the Office on Women's Health.

9 United States Department of Health and Human Services, Office on Women's Health. *National Breastfeeding Campaign Ad Council Materials.* Available at: http://www.womenshealth.gov/breast-feeding/government-programs/national-breastfeeding-campaign/adcouncil/ Accessed October 26, 2010. Reprinted by Permission of the Office on Women's Health.

10 United States Department of Health and Human Services, Office on Women's Health. *National Breastfeeding Campaign Ad Council Materials.* Available at: http://www.womenshealth.gov/breast-feeding/government-programs/national-breastfeeding-campaign/adcouncil/ Accessed October 26, 2010. Reprinted by Permission of the Office on Women's Health.

11 La Leche League International. *The Womanly Art of Breastfeeding. Seventh Revised Edition.* Schaumburg, IL: La Leche League International; 2003:6,339-349.

12 Meek JY, Editor. *American Academy of Pediatrics New Mother's Guide to Breastfeeding.* New York, NY: Bantam Books; 2002:6.

13 Meek JY, Editor. *American Academy of Pediatrics New Mother's Guide to Breastfeeding.* New York, NY: Bantam Books; 2002:8.

14 Meek JY, Editor. *American Academy of Pediatrics New Mother's Guide to Breastfeeding*. New York, NY: Bantam Books; 2002:8-9.

15 La Leche League International. *The Womanly Art of Breastfeeding. Seventh Revised Edition.* Schaumburg, IL: La Leche League International; 2003:341,344,374.

16 La Leche League International. *The Womanly Art of Breastfeeding. Seventh Revised Edition.* Schaumburg, IL: La Leche League International; 2003:6,342.

17 Meek JY, Editor. *American Academy of Pediatrics New Mother's Guide to Breastfeeding*. New York, NY: Bantam Books; 2002:7.

18 La Leche League International. *The Womanly Art of Breastfeeding. Seventh Revised Edition.* Schaumburg, IL: La Leche League International; 2003:6,368.

19 Armstrong J, Reilly JJ. Breastfeeding and lowering the risk of childhood obesity. *Lancet.* 2002;359:2003-2004.

20 Toschke AM, Vignerova J, Lhotska L, Osancova K, Koletzko B, von Kries R. Overweight and obesity in 6- to 14-year-old Czech children in 1991: Protective effect of breast feeding. *J Pediatr.* 2002;141;764-769.

21 Owen CG, Martin RM, Whincup PH, Smith GD, Cook DG. Effect of infant feeding on the risk of obesity across the life course: A quantitative review of published evidence. *Pediatrics.* 2005; 115:1367-1377.

22 Harder T, Bergmann R, Kallischnigg G, Plagemann A. Duration of breastfeeding and risk of overweight: A meta-analysis. *Am J Epidemiol.* 2005;162:397-403.

23 Weyermann M, Rothenbacher D, Brenner H. Duration of breastfeeding and risk of overweight in childhood: A prospective birth cohort study from Germany. *Int J Obes.* 2006;30:1281-1287.

24 von Kries R, Koletzko B, Sauerwald T, von Mutius E, Barnert D, Grunert V, von Voss H. Breast feeding and obesity: Cross sectional study. *BMJ.* 1999;319:147-150.

25 Gillman MW, Rifas-Shiman SL, Camargo CA, Berkey C, Frazier AL, Rockett HRH, Field AE, Colditz GA. Risk of overweight among adolescents who were breastfed as infants. *JAMA.* 2001;285:2461-2467.

26 Gillman MW, Rifas-Shiman SL, Camargo CA, Berkey C, Frazier AL, Rockett HRH, Field AE, Colditz GA. Risk of overweight among adolescents who were breastfed as infants. *JAMA.* 2001;285:2461-2467.

27 Meek JY, Editor. *American Academy of Pediatrics New Mother's Guide to Breastfeeding*. New York, NY: Bantam Books; 2002:183.

28 Meek JY, Editor. *American Academy of Pediatrics New Mother's Guide to Breastfeeding*. New York, NY: Bantam Books; 2002:7.

29 La Leche League International. *The Womanly Art of Breastfeeding. Seventh Revised Edition.* Schaumburg, IL: La Leche League International; 2003:6,356-359.

30 Meek JY, Editor. *American Academy of Pediatrics New Mother's Guide to Breastfeeding*. New York, NY: Bantam Books; 2002:5,7-8.

31 La Leche League International. *The Womanly Art of Breastfeeding. Seventh Revised Edition.* Schaumburg, IL: La Leche League International; 2003:6,352-353.

32 La Leche League International. *The Womanly Art of Breastfeeding. Seventh Revised Edition.* Schaumburg, IL: La Leche League International; 2003:6,359-363.

33 Bloch AM, Mimouni A, Mimouni D, Gdalevich M. Does breastfeeding protect against allergic rhinitis during childhood? A meta-analysis of prospective studies. *Acta Paediatr.* 2002; 91:275-279.

34 Friedman NJ, Zeiger RS. The role of breast-feeding in the development of allergies and asthma. *J Allergy Clin Immunol.* 2005;115:1238-1248.

35 La Leche League International. *The Womanly Art of Breastfeeding. Seventh Revised Edition.* Schaumburg, IL: La Leche League International; 2003:6,353-354.

36 La Leche League International. *The Womanly Art of Breastfeeding. Seventh Revised Edition.* Schaumburg, IL: La Leche League International; 2003:353-354.

37 Sadauskaite-Kuehne V, Ludvigsson J, Padaiga Ž, Jašinskienė E, and Samuelsson U. Longer breastfeeding is an independent protective factor against development of type 1 diabetes mellitus in childhood. *Diabetes/Metabolism Research and Reviews.* 2004; 20:150-157.

38 Owen CG, Martin RM, Whincup PH, Smith GD, Cook DG. Does breastfeeding influence risk of type 2 diabetes in later life? A quantitative analysis of published evidence. *Am J Clin Nutr.* 2006;84:1043-1054.

39 Singhal A. The early origins of atherosclerosis. *Adv Exp Med Biol.* 2009;646:51-58.

40 Owen CG, Whincup PH, Kaye SJ, Martin RM, Davey Smith G, Cook DG, Bergstrom E, Black S, Wadsworth ME, Fall CH, Freudenheim JL, Nie J, Huxley RR, Kolacek S, Leeson CP, Pearce MS, Raitakari OT, Lisinen I, Viikari JS, Ravelli AC, Rudnicka AR, Strachan DP, Williams SM. Does initial breastfeeding lead to lower blood cholesterol in adult life? A quantitative review of the evidence. *Am J Clin Nutr.* 2008;88:305-314.

41 Meek JY, Editor. *American Academy of Pediatrics New Mother's Guide to Breastfeeding.* New York, NY: Bantam Books; 2002:7.

42 Kwan ML, Buffler PA, Abrams B, Kiley VA. Breastfeeding and the risk of childhood leukemia: a meta-analysis. *Public Health Rep.* 2004; 119:521-535.

43 Meek JY, Editor. *American Academy of Pediatrics New Mother's Guide to Breastfeeding.* New York, NY: Bantam Books; 2002:5,7.

44 Freudenheim JL, Marshall JR, Graham S, Laughlin R, Vena JE, Elisa Bandera E, Muti P, Swanson M, Nemoto T. Exposure to breast milk in infancy and the risk of breast cancer. *Epidemiology.* 1994; 5:324-331.

45 Oddy WH, Peat JK, de Klerk NH. Maternal asthma, infant feeding, and the risk of asthma in childhood. *J Allergy Clin Immunol.* 2002;110:65-67.

46 Gdalevich M, Mimouni D, Mimouni M. Breast-feeding and the risk of bronchial asthma in childhood: A systematic review with meta-analysis of prospective studies. *J Pediatr.* 2001;139:261-266.

47 Gearry, RB, Richardson AK, Frampton CM, Dodgshun AJ, Barclay ML. Population-based cases control study of inflammatory bowel disease risk factors. *J Gastroenterol Hepatol.* 2010;25:325-333.

48 Barclay AR, Russell RK, Wilson ML, Gilmour WH, Satsangi J, Wilson DC. Systematic review: The role of breastfeeding in the development of pediatric inflammatory bowel disease. *J Pediatr.* 2009;155:421-426.

49 Meek JY, Editor. *American Academy of Pediatrics New Mother's Guide to Breastfeeding*. New York, NY: Bantam Books; 2002:7-8.

50 La Leche League International. *The Womanly Art of Breastfeeding. Seventh Revised Edition*. Schaumburg, IL: La Leche League International; 2003:354.

51 Vennemann MM, Bajanowski T, Brinkmann B, Jorch G, Yücesan K, Sauerland C, Mitchell ED, and the GeSID Study Group. Does breastfeeding reduce the risk of sudden infant death syndrome? *Pediatrics*.2009;123:e406-e410.

52 Schultz ST, Klonoff-Cohen HS, Wingard DL, Akshoomoff NA, Macera CA, Ji M, Bacher C. Breastfeeding, infant formula supplementation, and Autistic Disorder: The results of a parent survey. *Int Breastfeed J*. 2006;1:16.

53 Tanoue Y, Oda S. Weaning time of children with infantile autism. *J Autism Dev Disord*. 1989;19:425-434.

54 Meek JY, Editor. *American Academy of Pediatrics New Mother's Guide to Breastfeeding*. New York, NY: Bantam Books; 2002:9.

55 La Leche League International. *The Womanly Art of Breastfeeding. Seventh Revised Edition*. Schaumburg, IL: La Leche League International; 2003:6,365-367.

56 Meek JY, Editor. *American Academy of Pediatrics New Mother's Guide to Breastfeeding*. New York, NY: Bantam Books; 2002:9.

57 La Leche League International. *The Womanly Art of Breastfeeding. Seventh Revised Edition*. Schaumburg, IL: La Leche League International; 2003:6,365-367.

58 Kramer M, Aboud F, Mironova E, Vanilovich I, Platt RW, Matush L, Igumnov S, Fombonne E, Bogdanovich E, Ducruet T, Collet J-P, Chalmers B, Hodnett E, Davidovsky S, Skugarevsky O, Trofimovich O, Kozlova L, Shapiro S for the Promotion of Breastfeeding Intervention Trial (PROBIT) Study Group. Breastfeeding and child cognitive development: New evidence from a large randomized trial. *Arch Gen Psychiatry*. 2008;65:578-584.

59 Victora CG, Barros FC, Horta BL, Lima RC. Breastfeeding and school achievement in Brazilian adolescents. *Acta Paediatr*. 2005;94:1656-1660.

60 Horwood LJ, Fergusson DM. Breastfeeding and later cognitive and academic outcomes. *Pediatrics*. 1998;101:e9.

61 Mortensen EL, Michaelsen KF, Sanders SA, Reinisch JM. The association between duration of breastfeeding and adult intelligence. *JAMA*. 2002; 287:2365-2371.

62 Horwood LJ, Fergusson DM. Breastfeeding and later cognitive and academic outcomes. *Pediatrics*. 1998;101:e9.

63 Angelsen NK, Vik T, Jacobsen G, Bakketeig LS. Breast feeding and cognitive development at age 1 and 5 years. *Arch Dis Child*. 2001; 85:183-188.

64 La Leche League International. *The Womanly Art of Breastfeeding. Seventh Revised Edition*. Schaumburg, IL: La Leche League International; 2003:368.

65 Montgomery SM, Ehlin, A, Sacker A. Breast feeding and resilience against psychosocial stress. *Arch Dis Child*. 2006;91:990-994.

66 Meek JY, Editor. *American Academy of Pediatrics New Mother's Guide to Breastfeeding*. New York, NY: Bantam Books; 2002:10.

67 La Leche League International. *The Womanly Art of Breastfeeding. Seventh Revised Edition.* Schaumburg, IL: La Leche League International; 2003:6-7,377.

68 Meek JY, Editor. *American Academy of Pediatrics New Mother's Guide to Breastfeeding.* New York, NY: Bantam Books; 2002:9,10.

69 Meek JY, Editor. *American Academy of Pediatrics New Mother's Guide to Breastfeeding.* New York, NY: Bantam Books; 2002:9.

70 La Leche League International. *The Womanly Art of Breastfeeding. Seventh Revised Edition.* Schaumburg, IL: La Leche League International; 2003:6,21,76-77.

71 Meek JY, Editor. *American Academy of Pediatrics New Mother's Guide to Breastfeeding.* New York, NY: Bantam Books; 2002:9,10.

72 La Leche League International. *The Womanly Art of Breastfeeding. Seventh Revised Edition.* Schaumburg, IL: La Leche League International; 2003:6,387-388.

73 Meek JY, Editor. *American Academy of Pediatrics New Mother's Guide to Breastfeeding.* New York, NY: Bantam Books; 2002:10.

74 La Leche League International. *The Womanly Art of Breastfeeding. Seventh Revised Edition.* Schaumburg, IL: La Leche League International; 2003:7,379,382-383.

75 Wolf JH. Low breastfeeding rates and public health in the United States. *Am J Public Health.* 2003;93:2000-2008.

76 Schwarz EB, Ray RM, Stuebe AM, Allison MA, Ness RB, Freiberg MS, Cauley JA. Duration of lactation and risk factors for maternal cardiovascular disease. *Obstet Gynecol.* 2009;113:974-982.

77 Lee SY, Kim MT, Jee SH, Yang HP. Does long-term lactation protect premenopausal women against hypertension risk? A Korean women's cohort study. *Prev Med.* 2005;41:433-438.

78 Stuebe AM, Rich-Edwards JW, Willett WC, Manson JE, Michels KB. Duration of lactation and incidence of type 2 diabetes. *JAMA.* 2005;294:2601-2610.

79 Schwarz EB, Ray RM, Stuebe AM, Allison MA, Ness RB, Freiberg MS, Cauley JA. Duration of lactation and risk factors for maternal cardiovascular disease. *Obstet Gynecol.* 2009;113:974-982.

80 Stuebe AM, Rich-Edwards JW, Willett WC, Manson JE, Michels KB. Duration of lactation and incidence of type 2 diabetes. *JAMA.* 2005;294:2601-2610.

81 Mosca L, Banka CL, Benjamin EJ, Berra K, Bushnell C, Dolor RJ, Ganiats TG, Gomes AS, Gornik HL, Gracia C, Gulati M, Haan CK, Judelson DR, Keenan N, Kelepouris E, Michos ED, Newby LK, Oparil S, Ouyang P, Oz MC, Petitti D, Pinn VW, Redberg RF, Scott R, Sherif K, Smith SC Jr, Sopko G, Steinhorn RH, Stone NJ, Taubert KA, Todd BA, Urbina E, Wenger NK for the Expert Panel/Writing Group. Evidence-based guidelines for cardiovascular disease prevention in women: 2007 update. *Circulation.* 2007;115:1481-501.

82 Meek JY, Editor. *American Academy of Pediatrics New Mother's Guide to Breastfeeding.* New York, NY: Bantam Books; 2002:10.

83 La Leche League International. *The Womanly Art of Breastfeeding. Seventh Revised Edition.* Schaumburg, IL: La Leche League International; 2003:7,378.

84 Sjögren B, Widström AM, Edman G, Uvnaus-Moberg K. Changes in personality pattern during the first pregnancy and lactation. *J Psychosom Obstet Gynaecol.* 2000;21:31-38.

85 Groer MW. Differences between exclusive breastfeeders, formula-feeders, and controls: A study of stress, mood, and endocrine variables. *Biol Res Nurs*. 2005;7:106-117.

86 McKee MD, Zayas LH, Jankowski KRB. Breastfeeding intention and practice in an urban minority population: Relationship to maternal depressive symptoms and mother infant closeness. *J Reprod Infant Psychol*. 2004;22:167-181.

87 Meek JY, Editor. *American Academy of Pediatrics New Mother's Guide to Breastfeeding*. New York, NY: Bantam Books; 2002:10.

88 La Leche League International. *The Womanly Art of Breastfeeding. Seventh Revised Edition*. Schaumburg, IL: La Leche League International; 2003:375-376.

89 Meek JY, Editor. *American Academy of Pediatrics New Mother's Guide to Breastfeeding*. New York, NY: Bantam Books; 2002:11.

CHAPTER 4: HEALTHY EATING HABITS BEGIN EARLY

1 Nader PR, O'Brien M, Houts R, Bradley R, Belsky J, Crosnoe R, Friedman S, Mei Z, Susman EJ. Identifying risk for obesity in early childhood. *Pediatrics*. 2006;118:e594-e601.

2 Harrington JW, Nguyen VQ, Paulson JF, Garland R, Pasquinelli L, Lewis D. Identifying the "tipping point" age for overweight pediatric patients. *Clin Pediatr*. 2010;49:638-643.

3 Fox MK, Pac S, Devaney B, Jankowski L. Feeding Infants and Toddlers Study: What foods are infants and toddlers eating? *J Am Diet Assoc*. 2004;104(suppl 1):S22-S30.

4 Elliott CD. Sweet and salty: Nutritional content and analysis of baby and toddler foods. *J Public Health (Oxf)*. June 28, 2010 [Epub ahead of print]:1-8. Available at: http://jpubhealth.oxfordjournals.org/content/early/2010/06/28/pubmed.fdq037.full.pdf. Accessed January 5, 2011.

5 Skinner JD, Ziegler P, Pac S, Devaney B. Meal and snack patterns of infants and toddlers. *J Am Diet Assoc*. 2004;104:S65-S70.

6 Cornwell TB, McAlister AR. Alternative thinking about starting points of obesity: Development of child taste preferences. *Appetite*. 2011;56:428-439.

7 Nader PR, O'Brien M, Houts R, Bradley R, Belsky J, Crosnoe R, Friedman S, Mei Z, Susman EJ. Identifying risk for obesity in early childhood. *Pediatrics*. 2006;118:e594-e601.

8 Fox MK, Pac S, Devaney B, Jankowski L. Feeding Infants and Toddlers Study: What foods are infants and toddlers eating? *J Am Diet Assoc*. 2004;104(suppl 1):S22-S30.

9 Stang J. Improving the eating patterns of infants and toddlers. *J Am Diet Assoc*. 2006;106(suppl 1):S7-S9.

10 Taveras EM, Rifas-Shiman SL, Berkey CS, Rocket HR, Field AE, Frazier AL, Colditz GA, Gillman MW. Family dinner and adolescent overweight. *Obes Res*. 2005;13:900–906.

11 Peters R. *It's Never Too Soon to Discipline: A Low-Stress Program That Shows Parents How to Teach Good Behavior That Will Last a Lifetime*. New York, NY: St. Martin's Press; 1998: 85.

12 Fox MK, Pac S, Devaney B, Jankowski L. Feeding Infants and Toddlers Study: What foods are infants and toddlers eating? *J Am Diet Assoc*. 2004;104(suppl 1):S22-S30.

13 Stang J. Improving the eating patterns of infants and toddlers. *J Am Diet Assoc*. 2006;106(suppl 1):S7-S9

14 Cornwell TB, McAlister AR. Alternative thinking about starting points of obesity: Development of child taste preferences. *Appetite*. 2011;56:428-439.

15 American Academy of Pediatrics, Committee on Nutrition. Policy Statement: The use and misuse of fruit juice in pediatrics. *Pediatrics*. 2001;107:1210-1213.

16 Fox MK, Pac S, Devaney B, Jankowski L. Feeding Infants and Toddlers Study: What foods are infants and toddlers eating? *J Am Diet Assoc*. 2004;104(suppl 1):S22-S30.

17 Fox MK, Pac S, Devaney B, Jankowski L. Feeding Infants and Toddlers Study: What foods are infants and toddlers eating? *J Am Diet Assoc*. 2004;104(suppl 1):S22-30.

18 Fox MK, Pac S, Devaney B, Jankowski L. Feeding Infants and Toddlers Study: What foods are infants and toddlers eating? *J Am Diet Assoc*. 2004;104(suppl 1):S22-30.

19 Heird WC, Ziegler P, Reidy K, Briefel R. Current electrolyte intakes of infants and toddlers. *J Am Diet Assoc*. 2006;106(suppl 1):S43-S51.

20 Fox MK, Pac S, Devaney B, Jankowski L. Feeding Infants and Toddlers Study: What foods are infants and toddlers eating? *J Am Diet Assoc*. 2004;104(suppl 1):S22-S30.

21 Heird WC, Ziegler P, Reidy K, Briefel RR. Current electrolyte intakes of infants and toddlers. *J Am Diet Assoc*. 2006;106(suppl 1):S43-S51.

22 Fox MK, Reidy K, Novak T, Ziegler P. Sources of energy and nutrients in the diets of infants and toddlers. *J Am Diet Assoc*. 2006;106(suppl 1):S28-S42.

23 Stang J. Improving the eating patterns of infants and toddlers. *J Am Diet Assoc*. 2006;106(suppl 1):S7-S9

24 Fox MK, Reidy K, Novak T, Ziegler P. Sources of energy and nutrients in the diets of infants and toddlers. *J Am Diet Assoc*. 2006;106(suppl 1):S28-S42.

25 Stang J. Improving the eating patterns of infants and toddlers. *J Am Diet Assoc*. 2006;106(suppl 1):S7-S9

26 Skinner JD, Ziegler P, Pac S, Devaney B. Meal and snack patterns of infants and toddlers. *J Am Diet Assoc*. 2004;104:S65-S70.

27 Skinner JD, Ziegler P, Pac S, Devaney B. Meal and snack patterns of infants and toddlers. *J Am Diet Assoc*. 2004;104:S65-S70.

28 Stang J. Improving the eating patterns of infants and toddlers. *J Am Diet Assoc*. 2006;106(suppl 1):S7-S9

29 Briefel RR, Reidy K, Karwe V, Devaney B. Feeding Infants and Toddlers Study: Improvements needed in meeting infant feeding recommendations. *J Am Diet Assoc*. 2004;104(suppl 1):S31-S37.

30 Fox MK, Pac S, Devaney B, Jankowski L. Feeding Infants and Toddlers Study: What foods are infants and toddlers eating? *J Am Diet Assoc*. 2004;104(suppl 1): S22-S30.

31 Fox MK, Pac S, Devaney B, Jankowski L. Feeding Infants and Toddlers Study: What foods are infants and toddlers eating? *J Am Diet Assoc*. 2004;104(suppl 1):S22-S30.

32 Skinner JD, Ziegler P, Pac S, Devaney B. Meal and snack patterns of infants and toddlers. *J Am Diet Assoc*. 2004;104:S65-S70.

33 Fox MK, Pac S, Devaney B, Jankowski L. Feeding Infants and Toddlers Study: What foods are infants and toddlers eating? *J Am Diet Assoc.* 2004;104(suppl 1):S22-S30.

34 Heird WC, Ziegler P, Reidy K, Briefel RR. Current electrolyte intakes of infants and toddlers. *J Am Diet Assoc.* 2006;106(suppl 1):S43-S51.

35 Fox MK, Reidy K, Novak T, Ziegler P. Sources of energy and nutrients in the diets of infants and toddlers. *J Am Diet Assoc.* 2006;106(suppl 1):S28-S42.

36 Skinner JD, Ziegler P, Ponza M. Transitions in infants' and toddlers' beverage patterns. *J Am Diet Assoc.* 2004;104:S45-S50.

37 Skinner JD, Ziegler P, Pac S, Devaney B. Meal and snack patterns of infants and toddlers. *J Am Diet Assoc.* 2004;104:S65-S70.

38 Skinner JD, Ziegler P, Pac S, Devaney B. Meal and snack patterns of infants and toddlers. *J Am Diet Assoc.* 2004;104:S65-S70.

39 Fox MK, Pac S, Devaney B, Jankowski L. Feeding Infants and Toddlers Study: What foods are infants and toddlers eating? *J Am Diet Assoc.* 2004;104(suppl 1):S22-S30.

40 Skinner JD, Ziegler P, Pac S, Devaney B. Meal and snack patterns of infants and toddlers. *J Am Diet Assoc.* 2004;104:S65-S70.

41 Skinner JD, Ziegler P, Pac S, Devaney B. Meal and snack patterns of infants and toddlers. *J Am Diet Assoc.* 2004;104:S65-S70.

42 Stang J. Improving the eating patterns of infants and toddlers. *J Am Diet Assoc.* 2006;106(suppl 1):S7-S9

43 Skinner JD, Ziegler P, Pac S, Devaney B. Meal and snack patterns of infants and toddlers. J Am Diet Assoc. 2004;104:S65-S70.

44 Stang J. Improving the eating patterns of infants and toddlers. *J Am Diet Assoc.* 2006;106(suppl 1):S7-S9

45 Cornwell TB, McAlister AR. Alternative thinking about starting points of obesity: Development of child taste preferences. *Appetite.* 2011;56:428-439.

46 Cornwell TB, McAlister AR. Alternative thinking about starting points of obesity: Development of child taste preferences. *Appetite.* 2011;56:428-439.

47 Elliott CD. Sweet and salty: Nutritional content and analysis of baby and toddler foods. *J Public Health (Oxf).* June 28, 2010 [Epub ahead of print]:1-8. Available at: http://jpubhealth.oxfordjournals.org/content/early/2010/06/28/pubmed.fdq037.full.pdf. Accessed January 5, 2011.

48 Elliott CD. Sweet and salty: Nutritional content and analysis of baby and toddler foods. *J Public Health (Oxf).* June 28, 2010 [Epub ahead of print]:1-8. Available at: http://jpubhealth.oxfordjournals.org/content/early/2010/06/28/pubmed.fdq037.full.pdf. Accessed January 5, 2011.

49 Huh SY, Rifas-Shiman SL, Taveras EM, Oken E, Gillman MW. Timing of solid food introduction and risk of obesity in preschool-aged children. *Pediatrics.* 2011;127: e544-551.

50 Elliott CD. Sweet and salty: Nutritional content and analysis of baby and toddler foods. *J Public Health (Oxf).* June 28, 2010 [Epub ahead of print]:1-8. Available at: http://jpubhealth.oxfordjournals.org/content/early/2010/06/28/pubmed.fdq037.full.pdf. Accessed January 5, 2011.

51 Elliott CD. Sweet and salty: Nutritional content and analysis of baby and toddler foods. *J Public Health (Oxf)*. June 28, 2010 [Epub ahead of print]:1-8. Available at: http://jpubhealth.oxfordjournals. org/content/early/2010/06/28/pubmed.fdq037.full.pdf. Accessed January 5, 2011.

52 Daniels SR, Arnett DK, Eckel RH, Gidding SS, Hayman LL, Kumanyika S, Robinson TN, Scott BJ, St. Jeor S, Williams CL. Overweight in children and adolescents: Pathophysiology, consequences, prevention, and treatment. *Circulation*. 2005;111:1999-2012.

CHAPTER 5: A HEALTHY BREAKFAST

1 Cho S, Dietrich M, Brown C, Clark CA, Block G. The effect of breakfast type on total daily energy intake and body mass index: Results from the Third National Health and Nutrition Examination Survey (NHANES III). *J Am Coll Nutr*. 2003;22:296-302.

2 Rampersaud GC, Pereira MA, Girard BL, Adams J, Metzl JD. Breakfast habits, nutritional status, body weight, and academic performance in children and adolescents. *J Am Diet Assoc*. 2005;105:743-760.

3 Cho S, Dietrich M, Brown C, Clark CA, Block G. The effect of breakfast type on total daily energy intake and body mass index: Results from the Third National Health and Nutrition Examination Survey (NHANES III). *J Am Coll Nutr*. 2003;22:296-302.

4 Song WO, Chun OK, Obayashi S, Cho S, Chung CE. Is consumption of breakfast associated with body mass index in US adults? *J Am Diet Assoc*. 2005;105:1373-1382.

5 Rampersaud GC, Pereira MA, Girard BL, Adams J, Metzl JD. Breakfast habits, nutritional status, body weight, and academic performance in children and adolescents. *J Am Diet Assoc*. 2005;105:743-760.

6 Affenito SG, Thompson DR, Barton BA, Franko DL, Daniels SR, Obarzanek E, Schreiber GB, Striegel-Moore RH. Breakfast consumption by African-American and White adolescent girls correlates positively with calcium and fiber intake and negatively with body mass index. *J Am Diet Assoc*. 2005;105:938-945.

7 Affenito SG, Thompson DR, Barton BA, Franko DL, Daniels SR, Obarzanek E, Schreiber GB, Striegel-Moore RH. Breakfast consumption by African-American and White adolescent girls correlates positively with calcium and fiber intake and negatively with body mass index. *J Am Diet Assoc*. 2005;105:938-945.

8 Rampersaud GC, Pereira MA, Girard BL, Adams J, Metzl JD. Breakfast habits, nutritional status, body weight, and academic performance in children and adolescents. *J Am Diet Assoc*. 2005;105:743-760.

9 Haines J, Stang J. Promoting meal consumption among teens. *J Am Diet Assoc*. 2005;105:945-947.

10 Affenito SG, Thompson DR, Barton BA, Franko DL, Daniels SR, Obarzanek E, Schreiber GB, Striegel-Moore RH. Breakfast consumption by African-American and White adolescent girls correlates positively with calcium and fiber intake and negatively with body mass index. *J Am Diet Assoc*. 2005;105:938-945.

11 Siega-Riz AM, Popkin BM, Carson T. Trends in breakfast consumption for children in the United States from 1965-1991. *Am J Clin Nutr*. 1998;67(suppl):748S-756S.

12 Haines J, Stang J. Promoting meal consumption among teens. *J Am Diet Assoc*. 2005;105:945-947.

13 Rampersaud GC, Pereira MA, Girard BL, Adams J, Metzl JD. Breakfast habits, nutritional status, body weight, and academic performance in children and adolescents. *J Am Diet Assoc*. 2005;105:743-760.

14 Reddan J, Wahlstrom K, Reicks M. Children's perceived benefits and barriers in relation to eating breakfast in schools with or without Universal School Breakfast. *J Nutr Educ Behav.* 2002;34:47-52.

15 Cohen B, Evers S, Manske S, Bercovitz K, Edward HG. Smoking, physical activity and breakfast consumption among secondary school students in a southwestern Ontario community. *Can J Public Health.* 2003;94:41-44.

16 Reddan J, Wahlstrom K, Reicks M. Children's perceived benefits and barriers in relation to eating breakfast in schools with or without Universal School Breakfast. *J Nutr Educ Behav.* 2002;34:47-52.

17 Rampersaud GC, Pereira MA, Girard BL, Adams J, Metzl JD. Breakfast habits, nutritional status, body weight, and academic performance in children and adolescents. *J Am Diet Assoc.* 2005;105:743-760.

18 Rampersaud GC, Pereira MA, Girard BL, Adams J, Metzl JD. Breakfast habits, nutritional status, body weight, and academic performance in children and adolescents. *J Am Diet Assoc.* 2005;105:743-760.

19 Affenito SG, Thompson DR, Barton BA, Franko DL, Daniels SR, Obarzanek E, Schreiber GB, Striegel-Moore RH. Breakfast consumption by African-American and White adolescent girls correlates positively with calcium and fiber intake and negatively with body mass index. *J Am Diet Assoc.* 2005;105:938-945.

20 Rampersaud GC, Pereira MA, Girard BL, Adams J, Metzl JD. Breakfast habits, nutritional status, body weight, and academic performance in children and adolescents. *J Am Diet Assoc.* 2005;105:743-760.

21 Rampersaud GC, Pereira MA, Girard BL, Adams J, Metzl JD. Breakfast habits, nutritional status, body weight, and academic performance in children and adolescents. *J Am Diet Assoc.* 2005;105:743-760.

22 Barton BA, Eldridge AL, Thompson D, Affenito SG, Striegel-Moore RH, Franko DL, Albertson AM, Crockett SJ. The relationship of breakfast and cereal consumption to nutrient intake and body mass index: The National Heart, Lung, and Blood Institute Growth and Health Study. *J Am Diet Assoc.* 2005;105:1383-1389.

23 Affenito SG, Thompson DR, Barton BA, Franko DL, Daniels SR, Obarzanek E, Schreiber GB, Striegel-Moore RH. Breakfast consumption by African-American and White adolescent girls correlates positively with calcium and fiber intake and negatively with body mass index. *J Am Diet Assoc.* 2005;105:938-945.

24 Wilson NC, Parnell WR, Wohlers M, Shirley P. Eating breakfast and its impact on children's daily diet. *Nutrition & Dietetics.* 2006;63:15-20.

25 Nicklas TA, Bao W, Webber LS, Berenson GS. Breakfast consumption affects adequacy of total daily intake in children. *J Am Diet Assoc.* 1993;93:886-891.

26 Haines J, Stang J. Promoting meal consumption among teens. *J Am Diet Assoc.* 2005;105:945-947.

27 Albertson AM, Anderson GH, Crockett SJ, Goebel MT. Ready-to-eat cereal consumption: Its relationship with BMI and nutrient intake of children aged 4 to 12 years. *J Am Diet Assoc.* 2003;103:1613-1619.

28 Rampersaud GC, Pereira MA, Girard BL, Adams J, Metzl JD. Breakfast habits, nutritional status, body weight, and academic performance in children and adolescents. *J Am Diet Assoc.* 2005;105:743-760.

29 Rampersaud GC, Pereira MA, Girard BL, Adams J, Metzl JD. Breakfast habits, nutritional status, body weight, and academic performance in children and adolescents. *J Am Diet Assoc.* 2005;105:743-760.

30 Wyatt HR, Grunwald GK, Mosca CL, Klem ML, Wing RR, Hill JO. Long-term weight loss and breakfast in subjects in the National Weight Control Registry. *Obesity Research.* 2002;10:78-82.

31 Cho S, Dietrich M, Brown C, Clark CA, Block G. The effect of breakfast type on total daily energy intake and body mass index: Results from the Third National Health and Nutrition Examination Survey (NHANES III). *J Am Coll Nutr.* 2003;22:296-302.

32 Rampersaud GC, Pereira MA, Girard BL, Adams J, Metzl JD. Breakfast habits, nutritional status, body weight, and academic performance in children and adolescents. *J Am Diet Assoc.* 2005;105:743-760.

33 Affenito SG, Thompson DR, Barton BA, Franko DL, Daniels SR, Obarzanek E, Schreiber GB, Striegel-Moore RH. Breakfast consumption by African-American and White adolescent girls correlates positively with calcium and fiber intake and negatively with body mass index. *J Am Diet Assoc.* 2005;105:938-945.

34 Barton BA, Eldridge AL, Thompson D, Affenito SG, Striegel-Moore RH, Franko DL, Albertson AM, Crockett SJ. The relationship of breakfast and cereal consumption to nutrient intake and body mass index: The National Heart, Lung, and Blood Institute Growth and Health Study. *J Am Diet Assoc.* 2005;105:1383-1389.

35 Rampersaud GC, Pereira MA, Girard BL, Adams J, Metzl JD. Breakfast habits, nutritional status, body weight, and academic performance in children and adolescents. *J Am Diet Assoc.* 2005;105:743-760.

36 Fiore H, Travis S, Whalen A, Auinger P, Ryan S. Potentially protective factors associated with healthful body mass index in adolescents with obese and nonobese parents: A secondary data analysis of the Third National Health and Nutrition Examination Survey, 1988-1994. *J Am Diet Assoc.* 2006;106:55-64.

37 Affenito SG, Thompson DR, Barton BA, Franko DL, Daniels SR, Obarzanek E, Schreiber GB, Striegel-Moore RH. Breakfast consumption by African-American and White adolescent girls correlates positively with calcium and fiber intake and negatively with body mass index. *J Am Diet Assoc.* 2005;105:938-945.

38 Barton BA, Eldridge AL, Thompson D, Affenito SG, Striegel-Moore RH, Franko DL, Albertson AM, Crockett SJ. The relationship of breakfast and cereal consumption to nutrient intake and body mass index: The National Heart, Lung, and Blood Institute Growth and Health Study. *J Am Diet Assoc.* 2005;105:1383-1389.

39 Rampersaud GC, Pereira MA, Girard BL, Adams J, Metzl JD. Breakfast habits, nutritional status, body weight, and academic performance in children and adolescents. *J Am Diet Assoc.* 2005;105:743-760.

40 Fiore H, Travis S, Whalen A, Auinger P, Ryan S. Potentially protective factors associated with healthful body mass index in adolescents with obese and nonobese parents: A secondary data analysis of the Third National Health and Nutrition Examination Survey, 1988-1994. *J Am Diet Assoc.* 2006;106:55-64.

41 Jones SJ, Jahns L, Laraia BA, Haughton B. Lower risk of overweight in school-aged food insecure girls who participate in food assistance: Results from the Panel Study of Income Dynamics Child Development Supplement. *Arch Pediatr Adolesc Med.* 2003;157:780-784.

42 Haines J, Stang J. Promoting meal consumption among teens. *J Am Diet Assoc.* 2005;105:945-947.

43 Rampersaud GC, Pereira MA, Girard BL, Adams J, Metzl JD. Breakfast habits, nutritional status, body weight, and academic performance in children and adolescents. *J Am Diet Assoc.* 2005;105:743-760.

44 Haines J, Stang J. Promoting meal consumption among teens. *J Am Diet Assoc.* 2005;105:945-947.

45 Rampersaud GC, Pereira MA, Girard BL, Adams J, Metzl JD. Breakfast habits, nutritional status, body weight, and academic performance in children and adolescents. *J Am Diet Assoc.* 2005;105:743-760.

46 Albertson AM, Anderson GH, Crockett SJ, Goebel MT. Ready-to-eat cereal consumption: Its relationship with BMI and nutrient intake of children aged 4 to 12 years. *J Am Diet Assoc.* 2003;103:1613-1619.

47 Barton BA, Eldridge AL, Thompson D, Affenito SG, Striegel-Moore RH, Franko DL, Albertson AM, Crockett SJ. The relationship of breakfast and cereal consumption to nutrient intake and body mass index: The National Heart, Lung, and Blood Institute Growth and Health Study. *J Am Diet Assoc.* 2005;105:1383-1389.

48 Rampersaud GC, Pereira MA, Girard BL, Adams J, Metzl JD. Breakfast habits, nutritional status, body weight, and academic performance in children and adolescents. *J Am Diet Assoc.* 2005;105:743-760.

49 Wyon D, Abrahamsson L, Jartelius M, Fletcher R. An experimental study of the effects of energy intake at breakfast on the test performance of 10 year-old children in school. *Int J Food Sci Nutr.* 1997;48:5-12.

50 Murphy JM, Pagano M, Nachmani J, Sperling P, Kane S, Kleinman R. The relationship of school breakfast to psychosocial and academic functioning: Cross-sectional and longitudinal observations in an inner-city sample. *Arch Pediatr Adolesc Med.* 1998;152:899-907.

51 Murphy JM, Pagano M, Nachmani J, Sperling P, Kane S, Kleinman R. The relationship of school breakfast to psychosocial and academic functioning: Cross-sectional and longitudinal observations in an inner-city sample. *Arch Pediatr Adolesc Med.* 1998;152:899-907.

52 Rampersaud GC, Pereira MA, Girard BL, Adams J, Metzl JD. Breakfast habits, nutritional status, body weight, and academic performance in children and adolescents. *J Am Diet Assoc.* 2005;105:743-760.

53 Murphy JM, Pagano M, Nachmani J, Sperling P, Kane S, Kleinman R. The relationship of school breakfast to psychosocial and academic functioning: Cross-sectional and longitudinal observations in an inner-city sample. *Arch Pediatr Adolesc Med.* 1998;152:899-907.

54 Murphy JM, Drake JE, Weineke KM. Academics & Breakfast Connection Pilot: Final Report on New York's Classroom Breakfast Project. Albany, New York: Nutrition Consortium of New York State; 2005:12-13. Available at: http://www.nutritionconsortium.org/childnutrition/documents/FinalABCupdated.pdf. Accessed March 4, 2011.

55 Murphy JM, Drake JE, Weineke KM. Academics & Breakfast Connection Pilot: Final Report on New York's Classroom Breakfast Project. Albany, New York: Nutrition Consortium of New York State; 2005:12-13. Available at: http://www.nutritionconsortium.org/childnutrition/documents/FinalABCupdated.pdf. Accessed March 4, 2011.

56 Rampersaud GC, Pereira MA, Girard BL, Adams J, Metzl JD. Breakfast habits, nutritional status, body weight, and academic performance in children and adolescents. *J Am Diet Assoc.* 2005;105:743-760.

57 Albertson AM, Anderson GH, Crockett SJ, Goebel MT. Ready-to-eat cereal consumption: Its relationship with BMI and nutrient intake of children aged 4 to 12 years. *J Am Diet Assoc.* 2003;103:1613-1619.

58 Song WO, Chun OK, Kerver J, Cho S, Chung CE, Chung SJ. Ready-to-eat breakfast cereal consumption enhances milk and calcium intake in the US population. *J Am Diet Assoc.* 2006;106:1783-1789.

59 Rampersaud GC, Pereira MA, Girard BL, Adams J, Metzl JD. Breakfast habits, nutritional status, body weight, and academic performance in children and adolescents. *J Am Diet Assoc.* 2005;105:743-760.

60 Barton BA, Eldridge AL, Thompson D, Affenito SG, Striegel-Moore RH, Franko DL, Albertson AM, Crockett SJ. The relationship of breakfast and cereal consumption to nutrient intake and body mass index: The National Heart, Lung, and Blood Institute Growth and Health Study. *J Am Diet Assoc.* 2005;105:1383-1389.

61 Song WO, Chun OK, Kerver J, Cho S, Chung CE, Chung SJ. Ready-to-eat breakfast cereal consumption enhances milk and calcium intake in the US population. *J Am Diet Assoc.* 2006;106:1783-1789.

62 Barton BA, Eldridge AL, Thompson D, Affenito SG, Striegel-Moore RH, Franko DL, Albertson AM, Crockett SJ. The relationship of breakfast and cereal consumption to nutrient intake and body mass index: The National Heart, Lung, and Blood Institute Growth and Health Study. *J Am Diet Assoc.* 2005;105:1383-1389.

63 Song WO, Chun OK, Kerver J, Cho S, Chung CE, Chung SJ. Ready-to-eat breakfast cereal consumption enhances milk and calcium intake in the US population. *J Am Diet Assoc.* 2006;106:1783-1789.

64 Barton BA, Eldridge AL, Thompson D, Affenito SG, Striegel-Moore RH, Franko DL, Albertson AM, Crockett SJ. The relationship of breakfast and cereal consumption to nutrient intake and body mass index: The National Heart, Lung, and Blood Institute Growth and Health Study. *J Am Diet Assoc.* 2005;105:1383-1389.

65 Song WO, Chun OK, Kerver J, Cho S, Chung CE, Chung SJ. Ready-to-eat breakfast cereal consumption enhances milk and calcium intake in the US population. *J Am Diet Assoc.* 2006;106:1783-1789.

66 Albertson AM, Anderson GH, Crockett SJ, Goebel MT. Ready-to-eat cereal consumption: Its relationship with BMI and nutrient intake of children aged 4 to 12 years. *J Am Diet Assoc.* 2003;103:1613-1619.

67 Barton BA, Eldridge AL, Thompson D, Affenito SG, Striegel-Moore RH, Franko DL, Albertson AM, Crockett SJ. The relationship of breakfast and cereal consumption to nutrient intake and body mass index: The National Heart, Lung, and Blood Institute Growth and Health Study. *J Am Diet Assoc.* 2005;105:1383-1389.

68 Cho S, Dietrich M, Brown C, Clark CA, Block G. The effect of breakfast type on total daily energy intake and body mass index: Results from the Third National Health and Nutrition Examination Survey (NHANES III). *J Am Coll Nutr.* 2003;22:296-302.

69 Rampersaud GC, Pereira MA, Girard BL, Adams J, Metzl JD. Breakfast habits, nutritional status, body weight, and academic performance in children and adolescents. *J Am Diet Assoc.* 2005;105:743-760.

70 Rampersaud GC, Pereira MA, Girard BL, Adams J, Metzl JD. Breakfast habits, nutritional status, body weight, and academic performance in children and adolescents. *J Am Diet Assoc.* 2005;105:743-760.

71 Fox MK, Pac S, Devaney B, Jankowski L. Feeding Infants and Toddlers Study: What foods are infants and toddlers eating? *J Am Diet Assoc.* 2004;104(suppl 1):S22-S30.

CHAPTER 6: WHOLESOME LUNCHES & SNACKS

1 Story M. The third School Nutrition Dietary Assessment Study: Findings and policy implications for improving the health of U.S. children. *J Am Diet Assoc.* 2009;109(suppl 1):S7-S13.

2 Montanez Johner N. Evaluation's vital role in healthier school meals. *J Am Diet Assoc.* 2009;109(suppl 1):S18-S19.

3 Crepinsek MK, Gordon AR, McKinney PM, Condon EM, Wilson A. Meals offered and served in U.S. public schools: Do they meet nutrient standards? *J Am Diet Assoc.* 2009;109(suppl 1):S31-S43.

4 Miller C. A practice perspective on the third School Nutrition Dietary Assessment Study. *J Am Diet Assoc.* 2009;109(suppl 1):S14-S17.

5 Gordon AR, Cohen R, Crepinsek MK, Fox MK, Hall J, Zeidman E The third School Nutrition Dietary Assessment Study: Background and study design. *J Am Diet Assoc.* 2009;109(suppl 1):S20-S30.

6 Clark M, Fox MF. Nutritional quality of the diets of U.S. public school children and the role of school meal programs. *J Am Diet Assoc.* 2009;109(suppl 1):S44-S56.

7 Clark M, Fox MF. Nutritional quality of the diets of U.S. public school children and the role of school meal programs. *J Am Diet Assoc.* 2009;109(suppl 1):S44-S56.

8 Crepinsek MK, Gordon AR, McKinney PM, Condon EM, Wilson A. Meals offered and served in U.S. public schools: Do they meet nutrient standards? *J Am Diet Assoc.* 2009;109(suppl 1):S31-S43.

9 Crepinsek MK, Gordon AR, McKinney PM, Condon EM, Wilson A. Meals offered and served in U.S. public schools: Do they meet nutrient standards? *J Am Diet Assoc.* 2009;109(suppl 1):S31-S43.

10 Condon EM, Crepinsek MK, Fox MK. School meals: Types of foods offered to and consumed by children at lunch and breakfast. *J Am Diet Assoc.* 2009;109(suppl 1):S67-S78.

11 Story M. The third School Nutrition Dietary Assessment Study: Findings and policy implications for improving the health of U.S. children. *J Am Diet Assoc.* 2009;109(suppl 1):S7-S13.

12 Crepinsek MK, Gordon AR, McKinney PM, Condon EM, Wilson A. Meals offered and served in U.S. public schools: Do they meet nutrient standards? *J Am Diet Assoc.* 2009;109(suppl 1):S31-S43.

13 Story M. The third School Nutrition Dietary Assessment Study: Findings and policy implications for improving the health of U.S. children. *J Am Diet Assoc.* 2009;109(suppl 1):S7-S13.

14 Crepinsek MK, Gordon AR, McKinney PM, Condon EM, Wilson A. Meals offered and served in U.S. public schools: Do they meet nutrient standards? *J Am Diet Assoc.* 2009;109(suppl 1):S31-S43.

15 Briefel RR, Crespinsek MK, Cabili C, Wilson A, Gleason PM. School food environments and practices affect dietary behaviors of U.S. public school children. *J Am Diet Assoc.* 2009;109(suppl 1):S91-S107.

16 Briefel RR, Crespinsek MK, Cabili C, Wilson A, Gleason PM. School food environments and practices affect dietary behaviors of U.S. public school children. *J Am Diet Assoc.* 2009;109(suppl 1):S91-S107.

17 Story M. The third School Nutrition Dietary Assessment Study: Findings and policy implications for improving the health of U.S. children. *J Am Diet Assoc.* 2009;109(suppl 1):S7-S13.

18 Condon EM, Crepinsek MK, Fox MK. School meals: Types of foods offered to and consumed by children at lunch and breakfast. *J Am Diet Assoc.* 2009;109(suppl 1):S67-S78.

19 Condon EM, Crepinsek MK, Fox MK. School meals: Types of foods offered to and consumed by children at lunch and breakfast. *J Am Diet Assoc.* 2009;109(suppl 1):S67-S78.

20 Fox MK, Gordon A, Nogales R, Wilson A. Availability and consumption of competitive foods in U.S. public schools. *J Am Diet Assoc.* 2009:109(suppl 1);S57-S66.

21 Fox MK, Gordon A, Nogales R, Wilson A. Availability and consumption of competitive foods in U.S. public schools. *J Am Diet Assoc.* 2009:109(suppl 1);S57-S66.

22 Story M. The third School Nutrition Dietary Assessment Study: Findings and policy implications for improving the health of U.S. children. *J Am Diet Assoc.* 2009;109(suppl 1):S7-S13.

23 Briefel RR, Crespinsek MK, Cabili C, Wilson A, Gleason PM. School food environments and practices affect dietary behaviors of U.S. public school children. *J Am Diet Assoc.* 2009;109(suppl 1):S91-S107.

24 Fox MK, Gordon A, Nogales R, Wilson A. Availability and consumption of competitive foods in U.S. public schools. *J Am Diet Assoc.* 2009:109(suppl 1);S57-S66.

25 Fox MK, Gordon A, Nogales R, Wilson A. Availability and consumption of competitive foods in U.S. public schools. *J Am Diet Assoc.* 2009:109(suppl 1);S57-S66.

26 Fox MK, Gordon A, Nogales R, Wilson A. Availability and consumption of competitive foods in U.S. public schools. *J Am Diet Assoc.* 2009:109(suppl 1);S57-S66.

27 Story M. The third School Nutrition Dietary Assessment Study: Findings and policy implications for improving the health of U.S. children. *J Am Diet Assoc.* 2009;109(suppl 1):S7-S13.

28 Story M. The third School Nutrition Dietary Assessment Study: Findings and policy implications for improving the health of U.S. children. *J Am Diet Assoc.* 2009;109(suppl 1):S7-S13.

29 Briefel RR, Crespinsek MK, Cabili C, Wilson A, Gleason PM. School food environments and practices affect dietary behaviors of U.S. public school children. *J Am Diet Assoc.* 2009;109(suppl 1):S91-S107.

30 Briefel RR, Crespinsek MK, Cabili C, Wilson A, Gleason PM. School food environments and practices affect dietary behaviors of U.S. public school children. *J Am Diet Assoc.* 2009;109(suppl 1):S91-S107.

31 Fox MK, Gordon A, Nogales R, Wilson A. Availability and consumption of competitive foods in U.S. public schools. *J Am Diet Assoc.* 2009:109(suppl 1);S57-S66..

32 Fox MK, Hedley Dodd A, Wilson A, Gleason PM. Association between school food environment and practices and body mass index of U.S. public school children. *J Am Diet Assoc.* 2009;109(suppl 1):S108-S117.

33 Briefel RR, Wilson A, Gleason PM. Consumption of low-nutrient, energy-dense foods and beverages at school, home, and other locations among School Lunch participants and nonparticipants. *J Am Diet Assoc.* 2009;109(suppl 1):S79-S90.

34 Crepinsek MK, Gordon AR, McKinney PM, Condon EM, Wilson A. Meals offered and served in U.S. public schools: Do they meet nutrient standards? *J Am Diet Assoc.* 2009;109(suppl 1):S31-S43.

35 Condon EM, Crepinsek MK, Fox MK. School meals: Types of foods offered to and consumed by children at lunch and breakfast. *J Am Diet Assoc.* 2009;109(suppl 1):S67-S78.

36 Fox MK, Hedley Dodd A, Wilson A, Gleason PM. Association between school food environment and practices and body mass index of U.S. public school children. *J Am Diet Assoc.* 2009;109(suppl 1):S108-S117.

37 Anderson PM, Butcher KF. Reading, writing, and refreshments: Are school finances contributing to children's obesity? *J Hum Resources.* 2006;41:467-494.

38 Story M. The third School Nutrition Dietary Assessment Study: Findings and policy implications for improving the health of U.S. children. *J Am Diet Assoc.* 2009;109(suppl 1):S7-S13.

39 Forshee RA, Storey ML, Ginevan MD. A risk analysis model of the relationship between beverage consumption from school vending machines and risk of adolescent overweight. *Risk Analysis.* 2005;25:1121-1135.

40 Malik VS, Schulze MB, Hu FB. Intake of sugar-sweetened beverages and weight gain: a systematic review. *Am J Clin Nutr.* 2006;84:274-288.

41 Wiecha JL, Finkelstein D, Troped PJ, Fragala M, Peterson KE. School vending machine use an fast-food restaurant use are associated with sugar-sweetened beverage intake in youth. *J Am Diet Assoc.* 2006;106:1624-1630.

42 Briefel RR, Wilson A, Gleason PM. Consumption of low-nutrient, energy-dense foods and beverages at school, home, and other locations among School Lunch participants and nonparticipants. *J Am Diet Assoc.* 2009;109(suppl 1):S79-S90.

43 Briefel RR, Crespinsek MK, Cabili C, Wilson A, Gleason PM. School food environments and practices affect dietary behaviors of U.S. public school children. *J Am Diet Assoc.* 2009;109(suppl 1):S91-S107.

44 Briefel RR, Wilson A, Gleason PM. Consumption of low-nutrient, energy-dense foods and beverages at school, home, and other locations among School Lunch participants and nonparticipants. *J Am Diet Assoc.* 2009;109(suppl 1):S79-S90.

45 Briefel RR, Wilson A, Gleason PM. Consumption of low-nutrient, energy-dense foods and beverages at school, home, and other locations among School Lunch participants and nonparticipants. *J Am Diet Assoc.* 2009;109(suppl 1):S79-S90.

46 Nicklas TA, Morales M, Linares A, Yang SJ, Baranowski T, De Moor C, Berenson G. Children's meal patterns have changed over a 21-year period: The Bogalusa heart study. *J Am Diet Assoc.* 2004;104:753-761.

47 Condon EM, Crepinsek MK, Fox MK. School meals: Types of foods offered to and consumed by children at lunch and breakfast. *J Am Diet Assoc.* 2009;109(suppl 1):S67-S78.

48 Briefel RR, Crespinsek MK, Cabili C, Wilson A, Gleason PM. School food environments and practices affect dietary behaviors of U.S. public school children. *J Am Diet Assoc.* 2009;109(suppl 1):S91-S107.

49 Briefel RR, Crespinsek MK, Cabili C, Wilson A, Gleason PM. School food environments and practices affect dietary behaviors of U.S. public school children. *J Am Diet Assoc.* 2009;109(suppl 1):S91-S107.

50 Briefel RR, Wilson A, Gleason PM. Consumption of low-nutrient, energy-dense foods and beverages at school, home, and other locations among School Lunch participants and nonparticipants. *J Am Diet Assoc.* 2009;109(suppl 1):S79-S90.

CHAPTER 7: MORE FAMILY MEALS, LESS HAPPY MEALS

1 Paeratakul S, Ferdinand DP, Champagne CM, Ryan DH, Bray GA. Fast-food consumption among US adults and children: Dietary and nutrient intake profile. *J Am Diet Assoc.* 2003;103:1332-1338.

2 French SA, Lin BH, Guthrie JF. National trends in soft drink consumption among children and adolescents age 6 to 17 years: Prevalence, amounts, and sources, 1977/1978 to 1994/1998. *J Am Diet Assoc.* 2003;103:1326–1331.

3 Paeratakul S, Ferdinand DP, Champagne CM, Ryan DH, Bray GA. Fast-food consumption among US adults and children: Dietary and nutrient intake profile. *J Am Diet Assoc.* 2003;103:1332-1338.

4 Paeratakul S, Ferdinand DP, Champagne CM, Ryan DH, Bray GA. Fast-food consumption among US adults and children: Dietary and nutrient intake profile. *J Am Diet Assoc.* 2003;103:1332-1338.

5 Wiecha JL, Finkelstein D, Troped PJ, Fragala M, Peterson KE. School vending machine use and fast-food restaurant use are associated with sugar-sweetened beverage intake in youth. *J Am Diet Assoc.* 2006;106:1624-1630.

6 Nicklas TA, Morales M, Linares A, Yang SJ, Baranowski T, De Moor C, Berenson G. Children's meal patterns have changed over a 21-year period: The Bogalusa heart study. *J Am Diet Assoc.* 2004;104:753-761.

7 Ebbeling CB, Pawlak DB, Ludwig DS. Childhood obesity: public-health crisis, common sense cure. *Lancet.* 2002; 360:473-482

8 Nicklas TA, Demory-Luce D, Yang SJ, Baranowski T, Zakeri I, Berenson G. Children's food consumption patterns have changed over two decades (1973–1994): the Bogalusa heart study. *J Am Diet Assoc.* 2004;104:1127-1140.

9 Ebbeling CB, Pawlak DB, Ludwig DS. Childhood obesity: public-health crisis, common sense cure. *Lancet.* 2002; 360:473-482

10 French SA, Story M, Neumark-Sztainer D, Fulkerson JA, Hannan P. Fast food restaurant use among adolescents: associations with nutrient intake, food choices and behavioral and psychosocial variables. *Int J Obes Relat Metab Disord.* 2001;25:1823-1833.

11 Paeratakul S, Ferdinand DP, Champagne CM, Ryan DH, Bray GA. Fast-food consumption among US adults and children: Dietary and nutrient intake profile. *J Am Diet Assoc.* 2003;103:1332-1338.

12 Wiecha JL, Finkelstein D, Troped PJ, Fragala M, Peterson KE. School vending machine use an fast-food restaurant use are associated with sugar-sweetened beverage intake in youth. *J Am Diet Assoc.* 2006;106:1624-1630.

13 Nicklas TA, Morales M, Linares A, Yang SJ, Baranowski T, De Moor C, Berenson G. Children's meal patterns have changed over a 21-year period: The Bogalusa heart study. *J Am Diet Assoc.* 2004;104:753-761.

14 Paeratakul S, Ferdinand DP, Champagne CM, Ryan DH, Bray GA. Fast-food consumption among US adults and children: Dietary and nutrient intake profile. *J Am Diet Assoc.* 2003;103:1332-1338.

15 French SA, Story M, Neumark-Sztainer D, Fulkerson JA, Hannan P. Fast food restaurant use among adolescents: associations with nutrient intake, food choices and behavioral and psychosocial variables. *Int J Obes Relat Metab Disord.* 2001;25:1823-1833.

16 French SA, Lin BH, Guthrie JF. National trends in soft drink consumption among children and adolescents age 6 to 17 years: Prevalence, amounts, and sources, 1977/1978 to 1994/1998. *J Am Diet Assoc.* 2003;103:1326–1331.

17 Wiecha JL, Finkelstein D, Troped PJ, Fragala M, Peterson KE. School vending machine use an fast-food restaurant use are associated with sugar-sweetened beverage intake in youth. *J Am Diet Assoc.* 2006;106:1624-1630.

18 Council on Sports Medicine and Fitness and Council on School Health. Active healthy living: Prevention of childhood obesity through increased physical activity. *Pediatrics.* 2006;117:1834-1842.

19 Ebbeling CB, Pawlak DB, Ludwig DS. Childhood obesity: public-health crisis, common sense cure. *Lancet.* 2002; 360:473-482

20 Briefel RR, Wilson A, Gleason PM. Consumption of low-nutrient, energy-dense foods and beverages at school, home, and other locations among School Lunch participants and nonparticipants. *J Am Diet Assoc.* 2009;109(suppl 1):S79-S90.

21 Neumark-Sztainer D, Hannan PJ, Story M, Croll J, Perry C. Family meal patterns: Associations with socidodemographic characteristics and improved dietary intake among adolescents. *J Am Diet Assoc.* 2003;103:317-322.

22 Gillman MW, Rifas-Shiman SL, Frazier L, Rockett HRH, Camargo CA, Field AE, Berkey CS, Colditz GA. Family dinner and diet quality among older children and adolescents. *Arch Fam Med.* 2000;9:235-240.

23 Nicklas TA, Morales M, Linares A, Yang SJ, Baranowski T, De Moor C, Berenson G. Children's meal patterns have changed over a 21-year period: The Bogalusa heart study. *J Am Diet Assoc.* 2004;104:753-761.

24 Gillman MW, Rifas-Shiman SL, Frazier L, Rockett HRH, Camargo CA, Field AE, Berkey CS, Colditz GA. Family dinner and diet quality among older children and adolescents. *Arch Fam Med.* 2000;9:235-240.

25 Fulkerson JA, Neumark-Sztainer D, Story M. Adolescent and parent views of family meals. *J Am Diet Assoc.* 2006;106:526-532.

26 Taveras EM, Rifas-Shiman SL, Berkey CS, Rocket HRH, Field AE, Frazier AL, Colditz GA, Gillman MW. Family dinner and adolescent overweight. *Obes Res.* 2005;13:900-906.

27 Fulkerson JA, Neumark-Sztainer D, Story M. Adolescent and parent views of family meals. *J Am Diet Assoc.* 2006;106:526-532.

28 Gillman MW, Rifas-Shiman SL, Frazier L, Rockett HRH, Camargo CA, Field AE, Berkey CS, Colditz GA. Family dinner and diet quality among older children and adolescents. *Arch Fam Med.* 2000;9:235-240.

29 National Center on Addiction and Substance Abuse at Columbia University. *The Importance of Family Dinners IV.* New York, NY: National Center on Addiction and Substance Abuse; September 2007:13. Available at: http://www.casacolumbia.org/templates/publications_reports.aspx. Accessed on August 1, 2011.

30 Neumark-Sztainer D, Hannan PJ, Story M, Croll J, Perry C. Family meal patterns: Associations with socidodemographic characteristics and improved dietary intake among adolescents. *J Am Diet Assoc.* 2003;103:317-322.

31 Fulkerson JA, Neumark-Sztainer D, Story M. Adolescent and parent views of family meals. *J Am Diet Assoc.* 2006;106:526-532.

32 Neumark-Sztainer D, Hannan PJ, Story M, Croll J, Perry C. Family meal patterns: Associations with socidodemographic characteristics and improved dietary intake among adolescents. *J Am Diet Assoc.* 2003;103:317–322.

33 U.S. Department of Health and Human Services, Centers for Disease Control and Prevention. *State Indicator Report on Fruits and Vegetables, 2009.* Available at: http://www.fruitsandveggiesmatter.gov/downloads/StateIndicatorReport2009.pdf. Accessed August 1, 2011.

34 Taveras EM, Rifas-Shiman SL, Berkey CS, Rocket HRH, Field AE, Frazier AL, Colditz GA, Gillman MW. Family dinner and adolescent overweight. *Obes Res.* 2005;13:900-906.

35 Fulkerson JA, Neumark-Sztainer D, Story M. Adolescent and parent views of family meals. *J Am Diet Assoc.* 2006;106:526-532.

36 National Center on Addiction and Substance Abuse at Columbia University. *The Importance of Family Dinners V.* New York, NY: National Center on Addiction and Substance Abuse; September 2009:2. Available at: http://www.casacolumbia.org/templates/publications_reports.aspx. Accessed on August 1, 2011.

37 Cason KL. Family mealtimes: More than just eating together. *J Am Diet Assoc.* 2006;106:532-533.

38 Neumark-Sztainer D, Hannan PJ, Story M, Croll J, Perry C. Family meal patterns: Associations with sociodemographic characteristics and improved dietary intake among adolescents. *J Am Diet Assoc.* 2003;103:317-322.

39 Fulkerson JA, Neumark-Sztainer D, Story M. Adolescent and parent views of family meals. *J Am Diet Assoc.* 2006;106:526-532.

40 Neumark-Sztainer D, Hannan PJ, Story M, Croll J, Perry C. Family meal patterns: Associations with sociodemographic characteristics and improved dietary intake among adolescents. *J Am Diet Assoc.* 2003;103:317-322.

41 Fulkerson JA, Neumark-Sztainer D, Story M. Adolescent and parent views of family meals. *J Am Diet Assoc.* 2006;106:526-532.

42 Hammons AJ, Fiese BH. Is frequency of shared family meals related to the nutritional health of children and adolescents? *Pediatrics.* 2011;127:e1565-e1574.

43 Rampersaud GC, Pereira MA, Girard BL, Adams J, Metzl JD. Breakfast habits, nutritional status, body weight, and academic performance in children and adolescents. *J Am Diet Assoc.* 2005;105:743-760.

44 Neumark-Sztainer D, Hannan PJ, Story M, Croll J, Perry C. Family meal patterns: Associations with sociodemographic characteristics and improved dietary intake among adolescents. *J Am Diet Assoc.* 2003;103:317-322.

45 Rampersaud GC, Pereira MA, Girard BL, Adams J, Metzl JD. Breakfast habits, nutritional status, body weight, and academic performance in children and adolescents. *J Am Diet Assoc.* 2005;105:743-760.

46 Gillman MW, Rifas-Shiman SL, Frazier L, Rockett HRH, Camargo CA, Field AE, Berkey CS, Colditz GA. Family dinner and diet quality among older children and adolescents. *Arch Fam Med.* 2000;9:235-240.

47 Neumark-Sztainer D, Hannan PJ, Story M, Croll J, Perry C. Family meal patterns: Associations with sociodemographic characteristics and improved dietary intake among adolescents. *J Am Diet Assoc.* 2003;103:317-322.

48 Gillman MW, Rifas-Shiman SL, Frazier L, Rockett HRH, Camargo CA, Field AE, Berkey CS, Colditz GA. Family dinner and diet quality among older children and adolescents. *Arch Fam Med.* 2000;9:235-240.

49 Gillman MW, Rifas-Shiman SL, Frazier L, Rockett HRH, Camargo CA, Field AE, Berkey CS, Colditz GA. Family dinner and diet quality among older children and adolescents. *Arch Fam Med.* 2000;9:235-240.

50 Neumark-Sztainer D, Hannan PJ, Story M, Croll J, Perry C. Family meal patterns: Associations with sociodemographic characteristics and improved dietary intake among adolescents. *J Am Diet Assoc.* 2003;103:317-322.

51 Hammons AJ, Fiese BH. Is frequency of shared family meals related to the nutritional health of children and adolescents? *Pediatrics.* 2011;127:e1565-e1574.

52 Anderson SE, Whitaker RC. Household routines and obesity in U.S. preschool-aged children. *Pediatrics.* 2010;125:420-428.

53 Gable S, Chang Y, Krull JL. Television watching and frequency of family meals are predictive of overweight onset and persistence in a national sample of school-age children. *J Am Diet Assoc.* 2007;107:53-61.

54 Gillman MW, Rifas-Shiman SL, Frazier L, Rockett HRH, Camargo CA, Field AE, Berkey CS, Colditz GA. Family dinner and diet quality among older children and adolescents. *Arch Fam Med.* 2000;9:235-240.

55 Taveras EM, Rifas-Shiman SL, Berkey CS, Rocket HRH, Field AE, Frazier AL, Colditz GA, Gillman MW. Family dinner and adolescent overweight. *Obes Res.* 2005;13:900-906.

56 Hammons AJ, Fiese BH. Is frequency of shared family meals related to the nutritional health of children and adolescents? *Pediatrics.* 2011;127:e1565-e1574.

57 Fulkerson JA, Neumark-Sztainer D, Story M. Adolescent and parent views of family meals. *J Am Diet Assoc.* 2006;106:526-532.

58 Eisenberg ME, Olson RE, Neumark-Sztainer D, Story M, Bearinger LH. Correlations between family meals and psychosocial well-being among adolescents. *Arch Pediatr Adolesc Med.* 2004;158:792-796.

59 Fulkerson JA, Neumark-Sztainer D, Story M. Adolescent and parent views of family meals. *J Am Diet Assoc.* 2006;106:526-532.

60 Neumark-Sztainer D, Hannan PJ, Story M, Croll J, Perry C. Family meal patterns: Associations with sociodemographic characteristics and improved dietary intake among adolescents. *J Am Diet Assoc.* 2003;103:317-322.

61 Hammons AJ, Fiese BH. Is frequency of shared family meals related to the nutritional health of children and adolescents? *Pediatrics.* 2011;127:e1565-e1574.

62 Fulkerson JA, Neumark-Sztainer D, Story M. Adolescent and parent views of family meals. *J Am Diet Assoc.* 2006;106:526-532.

63 Eisenberg ME, Olson RE, Neumark-Sztainer D, Story M, Bearinger LH. Correlations between family meals and psychosocial well-being among adolescents. *Arch Pediatr Adolesc Med.* 2004;158:792-796

64 Morgan E, Kuykendall C. *What Every Child Needs: Meet Your Child's Nine Basic Needs for Love.* Grand Rapids, MI: Zondervan; 1997: 78-79. Reprinted by permission of MOPS International.

65 National Center on Addiction and Substance Abuse at Columbia University. *The Importance of Family Dinners VI.* New York, NY: National Center on Addiction and Substance Abuse; September 2010:2. Available at: http://www.casacolumbia.org/templates/publications_reports.aspx. Accessed on August 1, 2011.

66 National Center on Addiction and Substance Abuse at Columbia University. *The Importance of Family Dinners III*. New York, NY: National Center on Addiction and Substance Abuse; September 2006:i,9-10. Available at: http://www.casacolumbia.org/templates/publications_reports.aspx. Accessed on August 1, 2011.

67 National Center on Addiction and Substance Abuse at Columbia University. *The Importance of Family Dinners V.* New York, NY: National Center on Addiction and Substance Abuse; September 2009:8. Available at: http://www.casacolumbia.org/templates/publications_reports.aspx. Accessed on August 1, 2011.

68 Eisenberg ME, Olson RE, Neumark-Sztainer D, Story M, Bearinger LH. Correlations between family meals and psychosocial well-being among adolescents. *Arch Pediatr Adolesc Med.* 2004;158:792-796.

69 National Center on Addiction and Substance Abuse at Columbia University. *The Importance of Family Dinners VI*. New York, NY: National Center on Addiction and Substance Abuse; September 2010:i,5. Available at: http://www.casacolumbia.org/templates/publications_reports.aspx. Accessed on August 1, 2011.

70 National Center on Addiction and Substance Abuse at Columbia University. *The Importance of Family Dinners VI*. New York, NY: National Center on Addiction and Substance Abuse; September 2010:8. Available at: http://www.casacolumbia.org/templates/publications_reports.aspx. Accessed on August 1, 2011.

71 Eisenberg ME, Olson RE, Neumark-Sztainer D, Story M, Bearinger LH. Correlations between family meals and psychosocial well-being among adolescents. *Arch Pediatr Adolesc Med.* 2004;158:792-796.

72 Cason KL. Family mealtimes: More than just eating together. *J Am Diet Assoc.* 2006;106:532-533.

73 National Center on Addiction and Substance Abuse at Columbia University. *The Importance of Family Dinners VI*. New York, NY: National Center on Addiction and Substance Abuse; September 2010:4. Available at: http://www.casacolumbia.org/templates/publications_reports.aspx. Accessed on August 1, 2011.

74 Eisenberg ME, Olson RE, Neumark-Sztainer D, Story M, Bearinger LH. Correlations between family meals and psychosocial well-being among adolescents. *Arch Pediatr Adolesc Med.* 2004;158:792-796.

75 Gillman MW, Rifas-Shiman SL, Frazier L, Rockett HRH, Camargo CA, Field AE, Berkey CS, Colditz GA. Family dinner and diet quality among older children and adolescents. *Arch Fam Med.* 2000;9:235-240.

76 Fulkerson JA, Neumark-Sztainer D, Story M. Adolescent and parent views of family meals. *J Am Diet Assoc.* 2006;106:526-532.

77 Larson NI, Story M, Eisenberg ME, Neumark-Sztainer D. Food preparation and purchasing roles among adolescents: Associations with sociodemographic characteristics and diet quality. *J Am Diet Assoc.* 2006;106:211-218.

78 Cason KL. Family mealtimes: More than just eating together. *J Am Diet Assoc.* 2006;106:532-533.

CHAPTER 8: THE TRUTH ABOUT SWEETENED BEVERAGES

1 Nielsen SJ, Popkin BM. Changes in beverage intake between 1977 and 2001. *Am J Prev Med.* 2004;27:205-210.

2 Story M. The Third School Nutrition Dietary Assessment Study: Findings and policy implications for improving the health of US children. *J Am Diet Assoc.* 2009;109(suppl 1):S7-S13.

3 Ludwig DS, Peterson KE, Gortmaker SL. Relation between consumption of sugar-sweetened drinks and childhood obesity: A prospective, observational analysis. *Lancet.* 2001;357:505-508.

4 Skinner JD, Ziegler P, Ponza M. Transitions in infants' and toddlers' beverage patterns. *J Am Diet Assoc.* 2004;104:S45-S50.

5 O'Connor TM, Yang S, and Nicklas TA. Beverage intake among preschool children and its effect on weight status. *Pediatrics.* 2006;118:e1010-e1018.

6 French SA, Lin BH, Guthrie JF. National trends in soft drink consumption among children and adolescents age 6 to 17 years: Prevalence, amounts, and sources, 1977/1978 to 1994/1998. *JADA.* 2003;103:1326-1331.

7 Cavadini C, Siega-Riz AM, Popkin BM. US adolescent food intake trends from 1965 to 1996. *Arch Dis Child.* 2000;83:18-24

8 American Academy of Pediatrics, Committee on School Health. Policy Statement: Soft drinks in schools. *Pediatrics.* 2004;113:152-154.

9 Ludwig DS, Peterson KE, Gortmaker SL. Relation between consumption of sugar-sweetened drinks and childhood obesity: A prospective, observational analysis. *Lancet.* 2001;357:505-508.

10 French SA, Lin BH, Guthrie JF. National trends in soft drink consumption among children and adolescents age 6 to 17 years: Prevalence, amounts, and sources, 1977/1978 to 1994/1998. *JADA.* 2003;103:1326-1331.

11 French SA, Lin BH, Guthrie JF. National trends in soft drink consumption among children and adolescents age 6 to 17 years: Prevalence, amounts, and sources, 1977/1978 to 1994/1998. *JADA.* 2003;103:1326-1331.

12 Ludwig DS, Peterson KE, Gortmaker SL. Relation between consumption of sugar-sweetened drinks and childhood obesity: A prospective, observational analysis. *Lancet.* 2001;357:505-508.

13 Nicklas TA, Demory-Luce D, Yang SJ, Baranowski T, Zakeri I, Berenson G. Children's food consumption patterns have changed over two decades (1973–1994): The Bogalusa heart study. *J Am Diet Assoc.* 2004;104:1127-1140.

14 American Academy of Pediatrics, Committee on School Health. Policy Statement: Soft drinks in schools. *Pediatrics.* 2004;113:152-154.

15 Johnson RK, Appel LJ, Brands M, Howard BV, Lefevre M, Lustig RH, Sacks F, Steffen LM, Wylie-Rosett J. Dietary sugars intake and cardiovascular health: A Scientific Statement from the American Heart Association. *Circulation.* 2009;120:1011-1020.

16 Popkin BM, Nielsen SJ. The sweetening of the world's diet. *Obes Res.* 2003;11:1325–1332.

17 Ludwig DS, Peterson KE, Gortmaker SL. Relation between consumption of sugar-sweetened drinks and childhood obesity: A prospective, observational analysis. *Lancet.* 2001;357:505-508.

18 Malik VS, Schulze MB, Hu FB. Intake of sugar-sweetened beverages and weight gain: A systematic review. *Am J Clin Nutr.* 2006;84:274-288.

19 American Academy of Pediatrics, Committee on School Health. Policy Statement: Soft drinks in schools. *Pediatrics.* 2004;113:152-154.

20 Ludwig DS, Peterson KE, Gortmaker SL. Relation between consumption of sugar-sweetened drinks and childhood obesity: A prospective, observational analysis. *Lancet.* 2001;357:505-508.

21 Story M. The Third School Nutrition Dietary Assessment Study: Findings and policy implications for improving the health of US children. *J Am Diet Assoc.* 2009;109(suppl 1):S7-S13.

22 American Academy of Pediatrics, Committee on School Health. Policy Statement: Soft drinks in schools. *Pediatrics.* 2004;113:152-154.

23 Ludwig DS, Peterson KE, Gortmaker SL. Relation between consumption of sugar-sweetened drinks and childhood obesity: A prospective, observational analysis. *Lancet.* 2001;357:505-508.

24 Ebbeling CB, Pawlak DB, Ludwig DS. Childhood obesity: Public-health crisis, common sense cure. *Lancet.* 2002;360:473-482.

25 Striegel-Moore RH, Thompson D, Affenito SG, Franko DL, Obarzanek E, Barton BA, Schreiber GB. Daniels SR, Schmidt M, Crawford PB. Correlates of beverage intake in adolescent girls: The National Heart Lung and Blood Institute Growth and Health Study. *J Pediatr.* 2006;148:183–187.

26 O'Connor TM, Yang S, and Nicklas TA. Beverage intake among preschool children and its effect on weight status. *Pediatrics.* 2006;118:e1010-e1018.

27 Nicklas TA, Demory-Luce D, Yang SJ, Baranowski T, Zakeri I, Berenson G. Children's food consumption patterns have changed over two decades (1973–1994): The Bogalusa heart study. *J Am Diet Assoc.* 2004;104:1127-1140.

28 Malik VS, Schulze MB, Hu FB. Intake of sugar-sweetened beverages and weight gain: A systematic review. *Am J Clin Nutr.* 2006;84:274-288.

29 Malik VS, Schulze MB, Hu FB. Intake of sugar-sweetened beverages and weight gain: A systematic review. *Am J Clin Nutr.* 2006;84:274-288.

30 Malik VS, Schulze MB, Hu FB. Intake of sugar-sweetened beverages and weight gain: A systematic review. *Am J Clin Nutr.* 2006;84:274-288.

31 Troiano RP, Breifel RB, Carroll MD, Bialostosky K. Energy and fat intakes of children and adolescents in the United States: Data from the National Health and Nutrition Surveys. *Am J Clin Nutr.* 2000;72(suppl):1343S-1353S.

32 Malik VS, Schulze MB, Hu FB. Intake of sugar-sweetened beverages and weight gain: A systematic review. *Am J Clin Nutr.* 2006;84:274-288.

33 Welsh JA, Cogswell ME, Rogers S, Rockett H, Mei Z, Grummer-Strawn LM. Overweight among low-income preschool children associated with the consumption of sweet drinks: Missouri, 1999-2002. *Pediatrics.* 2005;115:e223-e229.

34 Malik VS, Schulze MB, Hu FB. Intake of sugar-sweetened beverages and weight gain: A systematic review. *Am J Clin Nutr.* 2006;84:274-288.

35 Nicklas TA, Yang SJ, Baranowski T, Zakeri I, Berenson G. Eating patterns and obesity in children. The Bogalusa Heart Study. *Am J Prev Med.* 2003;25:9-16.

36 Malik VS, Schulze MB, Hu FB. Intake of sugar-sweetened beverages and weight gain: A systematic review. *Am J Clin Nutr.* 2006;84:274-288.

37 Ebbeling CB, Feldman HA, Osganian, Stavroula SK, Chomitz VR, Ellenbogen SJ, Ludwig DS. Effects of decreasing sugar-sweetened beverage consumption on body weight in adolescents: A randomized, controlled pilot study. *Pediatrics.* 2006;117:673-680.

38 Ludwig DS, Peterson KE, Gortmaker SL. Relation between consumption of sugar-sweetened drinks and childhood obesity: A prospective, observational analysis. *Lancet.* 2001;357:505-508.

39 Striegel-Moore RH, Thompson D, Affenito SG, Franko DL, Obarzanek E, Barton BA, Schreiber GB. Daniels SR, Schmidt M, Crawford PB. Correlates of beverage intake in adolescent girls: The National Heart Lung and Blood Institute Growth and Health Study. *J Pediatr.* 2006;148:183–187.

40 American Academy of Pediatrics, Committee on School Health. Policy Statement: Soft drinks in schools. *Pediatrics.* 2004;113:152-154.

41 O'Connor TM, Yang S, and Nicklas TA. Beverage intake among preschool children and its effect on weight status. *Pediatrics.* 2006;118:e1010-e1018.

42 Skinner JD, Ziegler P, Ponza M. Transitions in infants' and toddlers' beverage patterns. *J Am Diet Assoc.* 2004;104:S45-S50.

43 Malik VS, Schulze MB, Hu FB. Intake of sugar-sweetened beverages and weight gain: A systematic review. *Am J Clin Nutr.* 2006;84:274-288.

44 Striegel-Moore RH, Thompson D, Affenito SG, Franko DL, Obarzanek E, Barton BA, Schreiber GB. Daniels SR, Schmidt M, Crawford PB. Correlates of beverage intake in adolescent girls: The National Heart Lung and Blood Institute Growth and Health Study. *J Pediatr.* 2006;148:183–187.

45 American Academy of Pediatrics, Committee on School Health. Policy Statement: Soft drinks in schools. *Pediatrics.* 2004;113:152-154.

46 American Academy of Pediatrics, Committee on School Health. Policy Statement: Soft drinks in schools. *Pediatrics.* 2004;113:152-154.

47 Troiano RP, Breifel RB, Carroll MD, Bialostosky K. Energy and fat intakes of children and adolescents in the United States: Data from the National Health and Nutrition Surveys. *Am J Clin Nutr.* 2000;72(suppl):1343S-1353S.

48 French SA, Lin BH, Guthrie JF. National trends in soft drink consumption among children and adolescents age 6 to 17 years: Prevalence, amounts, and sources, 1977/1978 to 1994/1998. *JADA.* 2003;103:1326-1331.

49 O'Connor TM, Yang S, and Nicklas TA. Beverage intake among preschool children and its effect on weight status. *Pediatrics.* 2006;118:e1010-e1018.

50 French SA, Lin BH, Guthrie JF. National trends in soft drink consumption among children and adolescents age 6 to 17 years: Prevalence, amounts, and sources, 1977/1978 to 1994/1998. *JADA.* 2003;103:1326-1331.

51 American Academy of Pediatrics, Committee on School Health. Policy Statement: Soft drinks in schools. *Pediatrics.* 2004;113:152-154.

52 French SA, Lin BH, Guthrie JF. National trends in soft drink consumption among children and adolescents age 6 to 17 years: Prevalence, amounts, and sources, 1977/1978 to 1994/1998. *JADA.* 2003;103:1326-1331.

53 Malik VS, Schulze MB, Hu FB. Intake of sugar-sweetened beverages and weight gain: A systematic review. *Am J Clin Nutr.* 2006;84:274-288.

54 American Academy of Pediatrics, Committee on School Health. Policy Statement: Soft drinks in schools. *Pediatrics.* 2004;113:152-154.

55 Schulze MB, Manson JE, Ludwig DS, et al. Sugar-sweetened beverages, weight gain, and incidence of type 2 diabetes in young and middle-aged women. *JAMA.* 2004;292:927-934.

56 American Academy of Pediatrics, Committee on Nutrition. Policy Statement: The use and misuse of fruit juice in pediatrics. *Pediatrics.* 2001;107:1210-1213.

57 American Academy of Pediatrics, Committee on Nutrition. Policy Statement: The use and misuse of fruit juice in pediatrics. *Pediatrics.* 2001;107:1210-1213.

58 Schulze MB, Manson JE, Ludwig DS, et al. Sugar-sweetened beverages, weight gain, and incidence of type 2 diabetes in young and middle-aged women. *JAMA.* 2004;292:927-934.

59 Malik VS, Schulze MB, Hu FB. Intake of sugar-sweetened beverages and weight gain: A systematic review. *Am J Clin Nutr.* 2006;84:274-288.

60 American Academy of Pediatrics, Committee on Nutrition. Policy Statement: The use and misuse of fruit juice in pediatrics. *Pediatrics.* 2001;107:1210-1213.

61 American Academy of Pediatrics, Committee on Nutrition. Policy Statement: The use and misuse of fruit juice in pediatrics. *Pediatrics.* 2001;107:1210-1213.

62 American Academy of Pediatrics, Committee on Nutrition. Policy Statement: The use and misuse of fruit juice in pediatrics. *Pediatrics.* 2001;107:1210-1213.

63 O'Connor TM, Yang S, and Nicklas TA. Beverage intake among preschool children and its effect on weight status. *Pediatrics.* 2006;118:e1010-e1018.

64 U.S. Department of Agriculture, U.S. Department of Health and Human Services. *Dietary Guidelines for Americans, 2010. Seventh Edition.* Washington, DC: U.S. Government Printing Office; 2010:78-80. Available at http://www.DietaryGuidelines.gov. Accessed: June 15, 2010.

65 Dietz, WH. Sugar-sweetened beverages, milk intake, and obesity in children and adolescents. *J Pediatr.* 2006;148:152-154.

66 Skinner JD, Ziegler P, Ponza M. Transitions in infants' and toddlers' beverage patterns. *J Am Diet Assoc.* 2004;104:S45-S50.

CHAPTER 9: ESTABLISHING PHYSICAL ACTIVITY HABITS EARLY

1 American Academy of Pediatrics, Committee on Nutrition. Policy Statement: Prevention of pediatric overweight and obesity. *Pediatrics.* 2003;112;424-430.

2 Council on Sports Medicine and Fitness and Council on School Health. Active healthy living: Prevention of childhood obesity through increased physical activity. *Pediatrics.* 2006;117:1834-1842.

3 Centers for Disease Control and Prevention. Surveillance of certain health behaviors among states and selected local areas: Behavioral Risk Factor Surveillance System, United States, 2007. *MMWR Surveill Summ.* 2010;59:4-5.

4 Ebbeling CB, Pawlak DB, Ludwig DS. Childhood obesity: Public-health crisis, common sense cure. *Lancet.* 2002;360:473-482.

5 Council on Sports Medicine and Fitness and Council on School Health. Active healthy living: Prevention of childhood obesity through increased physical activity. *Pediatrics.* 2006;117:1834-1842.

6 Centers for Disease Control and Prevention. Youth risk behavior surveillance: United States, 2009. *MMWR Surveill Summ.* 2010;59:25-26.

7 Lee SM, Burgeson CR, Fulton JE, Spain CG. Physical education and physical activity: Results from the School Health Policies and Programs Study 2006. *J Sch Health.* 2007;77:435-463.

8 American Academy of Pediatrics, Committee on Nutrition. Policy Statement: Prevention of pediatric overweight and obesity. *Pediatrics.* 2003;112;424-430.

9 Ebbeling CB, Pawlak DB, Ludwig DS. Childhood obesity: Public-health crisis, common sense cure. *Lancet.* 2002;360:473-482.

10 American Academy of Pediatrics, Committee on Nutrition. Policy Statement: Prevention of pediatric overweight and obesity. *Pediatrics.* 2003;112;424-430.

11 Centers for Disease Control and Prevention. Youth risk behavior surveillance: United States, 2009. *MMWR Surveill Summ.* 2010;59:34.

12 Lee SM, Burgeson CR, Fulton JE, Spain CG. Physical education and physical activity: Results from the School Health Policies and Programs Study 2006. *J Sch Health.* 2007;77:435-463.

13 Ebbeling CB, Pawlak DB, Ludwig DS. Childhood obesity: Public-health crisis, common sense cure. *Lancet.* 2002;360:473-482.

14 Council on Sports Medicine and Fitness and Council on School Health. Active healthy living: Prevention of childhood obesity through increased physical activity. *Pediatrics.* 2006;117:1834-1842.

15 Council on Sports Medicine and Fitness and Council on School Health. Active healthy living: Prevention of childhood obesity through increased physical activity. *Pediatrics.* 2006;117:1834-1842.

16 Lee SM, Burgeson CR, Fulton JE, Spain CG. Physical education and physical activity: Results from the School Health Policies and Programs Study 2006. *J Sch Health.* 2007;77:435-463.

17 U.S. Department of Health and Human Services, Centers for Disease Control and Prevention, National Center for Health Statistics. *Health, United States, 2005, With Chartbook on Trends in the Health of Americans.* Hyattsville, Maryland: National Center for Health Statistics; November 2005:38. Available at: http://www.ncbi.nlm.nih.gov/books/NBK20990/. Accessed February 9, 2011.

18 U.S. Department of Health and Human Services. *2008 Physical Activity Guidelines for Americans.* Washington, D.C.: U.S Department of Health and Human Services; October 2008:7-14. Available at: http://health.gov/paguidelines/guidelines/default.aspx. Accessed February 8, 2011.

19 U.S. Department of Health and Human Services, Centers for Disease Control and Prevention, National Center for Health Statistics. *Health, United States, 2005, With Chartbook on Trends in the Health of Americans.* Hyattsville, Maryland: National Center for Health Statistics; November 2005:38. Available at: http://www.ncbi.nlm.nih.gov/books/NBK20990/. Accessed February 9, 2011.

20 U.S. Department of Health and Human Services. *2008 Physical Activity Guidelines for Americans.* Washington, D.C.: U.S Department of Health and Human Services; October 2008:7-14. Available at: http://health.gov/paguidelines/guidelines/default.aspx. Accessed February 8, 2011.

21 Ralph S. Paffenbarger RS, Hyde R, Wing AL, Hsieh C-C. Physical activity, all-cause mortality, and longevity of college alumni. *N Engl J Med.* 1986; 314:605-613.

22 Council on Sports Medicine and Fitness and Council on School Health. Active healthy living: Prevention of childhood obesity through increased physical activity. *Pediatrics.* 2006;117:1834-1842.

23 Lee SM, Burgeson CR, Fulton JE, Spain CG. Physical education and physical activity: Results from the School Health Policies and Programs Study 2006. *J Sch Health.* 2007;77:435-463.

24 Ebbeling CB, Pawlak DB, Ludwig DS. Childhood obesity: Public-health crisis, common sense cure. *Lancet.* 2002;360:473-482.

25 Andersen RE, Crespo CJ, Bartlett SJ, Cheskin LJ, Pratt M. Relationship of physical activity and television watching with body weight and level of fatness among children: Results from the Third National Health and Nutrition Examination Survey. *JAMA.* 1998;279:938-942..

26 Robinson TN, Killen JD, Kraemer HC, Wilson DM, Matheson DM, Haskell WL, Pruitt LA, Powell TM, Owens AS, Thompson NS, Flint-Moore NM, Davis GJ, Emig KA, Brown RT, Rochon J, Green S, Varady A. Dance and reducing television viewing to prevent weight gain in African-American girls: The Stanford GEMS pilot study. *Ethn Dis.* 2003;13:S65-77.

27 American Academy of Pediatrics, Committee on Nutrition. Policy Statement: Prevention of pediatric overweight and obesity. *Pediatrics.* 2003;112;424-430.

28 Council on Sports Medicine and Fitness and Council on School Health. Active healthy living: Prevention of childhood obesity through increased physical activity. *Pediatrics.* 2006;117:1834-1842.

29 U.S. Department of Health and Human Services, Centers for Disease Control and Prevention, National Center for Health Statistics. *Health, United States, 2005, With Chartbook on Trends in the Health of Americans.* Hyattsville, Maryland: National Center for Health Statistics; November 2005:38. Available at: http://www.ncbi.nlm.nih.gov/books/NBK20990/. Accessed February 9, 2011.

30 Lee SM, Burgeson CR, Fulton JE, Spain CG. Physical education and physical activity: Results from the School Health Policies and Programs Study 2006. *J Sch Health.* 2007;77:435-463.

31 O'Connor TM, Yang S, and Nicklas TA. Beverage intake among preschool children and its effect on weight status. *Pediatrics.* 2006;118:e1010-e1018.

32 U.S. Department of Health and Human Services, Centers for Disease Control and Prevention, National Center for Health Statistics. *Health, United States, 2005, With Chartbook on Trends in the Health of Americans.* Hyattsville, Maryland: National Center for Health Statistics; November 2005:38. Available at: http://www.ncbi.nlm.nih.gov/books/NBK20990/. Accessed February 9, 2011.

33 Lee SM, Burgeson CR, Fulton JE, Spain CG. Physical education and physical activity: Results from the School Health Policies and Programs Study 2006. *J Sch Health.* 2007;77:435-463.

34 U.S. Department of Health and Human Services. *2008 Physical Activity Guidelines for Americans.* Washington, D.C.: U.S Department of Health and Human Services; October 2008: 21-23. Available at: http://health.gov/paguidelines/guidelines/default.aspx. Accessed February 8, 2011.

35 Haskell WL, Lee I-M, Pate RR, Powell KE, Blair SN, Franklin BA, Macera CA, Heath GW, Thompson PD, Bauman A. Physical activity and public health: Updated recommendation for adults from the American College of Sports Medicine and the American Heart Association. *Med Sci Sports Exerc.* 2007;39:1423–1434.

36 U.S. Department of Health and Human Services. *2008 Physical Activity Guidelines for Americans.* Washington, D.C.: U.S Department of Health and Human Services; October 2008:16. Available at: http://health.gov/paguidelines/guidelines/default.aspx. Accessed February 8, 2011.

37 U.S. Department of Health and Human Services. *2008 Physical Activity Guidelines for Americans.* Washington, D.C.: U.S Department of Health and Human Services; October 2008:16-17. Available at: http://health.gov/paguidelines/guidelines/default.aspx. Accessed February 8, 2011.

38 U.S. Department of Agriculture and U.S. Department of Health and Human Services. *2010 Dietary Guidelines for Americans, 7th Edition.* Washington, D.C.: U.S. Government Printing Office; December 2010:17. Available at: http://www.cnpp.usda.gov/DGAs2010-PolicyDocument.htm. Accessed February 8, 2011.

39 Daniels SR, Arnett DK, Eckel RH, Gidding SS, Hayman LL, Kumanyika S, Robinson TN, Scott BJ, St. Jeor S, Williams CL. Overweight in children and adolescents: Pathophysiology, consequences, prevention, and treatment. *Circulation.* 2005;111:1999-2012.

40 Cooper AR, Andersen LB, Wedderkopp N, Page AS, Froberg K. Physical activity levels of children who walk, cycle, or are driven to school. *Am J Prev Med.* 2005;29:179-184.

41 Sirard JR, Slater ME. Walking and bicycling to School: A review. *AJLM.* 2008;2:372-396.

42 Daniels SR, Arnett DK, Eckel RH, Gidding SS, Hayman LL, Kumanyika S, Robinson TN, Scott BJ, St. Jeor S, Williams CL. Overweight in children and adolescents: Pathophysiology, consequences, prevention, and treatment. *Circulation.* 2005;111:1999-2012.

43 Morgan E, Kuykendall C. *What Every Child Needs: Meet Your Child's Nine Basic Needs for Love.* Grand Rapids, MI: Zondervan; 1997:184. Reprinted by Permission of MOPS International.

44 Lakes KD, Hoyt WT. Promoting self-regulation through school-based martial arts training. *J Appl Dev Psychol.* 2004;25: 283-302.

CHAPTER 10: TOO MUCH SCREEN TIME

1 Rideout VJ, Foehr UG, Roberts DF. *Generation M²: Media in the Lives of 8- to 18- Year Olds.* Menlo Park, CA: The Henry J. Kaiser Family Foundation; 2010:9.

2 Roberts DF, Foehr UG, Rideout VJ, Brodie M. *Kids and Media at the New Millennium: A Comprehensive National Analysis of Children's Media Use.* Menlo Park, CA: The Henry J Kaiser Family Foundation; 1999:5, 23.

3 Rideout VJ, Foehr UG, Roberts DF. *Generation M²: Media in the Lives of 8- to 18-Year Olds.* Menlo Park, CA: The Henry J. Kaiser Family Foundation; 2010: 2.

4 Rideout VJ, Foehr UG, Roberts DF. *Generation M²: Media in the Lives of 8- to 18-Year Olds.* Menlo Park, CA: The Henry J. Kaiser Family Foundation; 2010:11.

5 Rideout VJ, Foehr UG, Roberts DF. *Generation M²: Media in the Lives of 8- to 18-Year Olds.* Menlo Park, CA: The Henry J. Kaiser Family Foundation; 2010:2.

6 Rideout VJ, Foehr UG, Roberts DF. *Generation M²: Media in the Lives of 8- to 18-Year Olds.* Menlo Park, CA: The Henry J. Kaiser Family Foundation; 2010:5.

7 Roberts DF, Foehr UG, Rideout VJ, Brodie M. *Kids and Media at the New Millennium: A Comprehensive National Analysis of Children's Media Use.* Menlo Park, CA: The Henry J Kaiser Family Foundation; 1999:21.

8 Rideout VJ, Foehr UG, Roberts DF. *Generation M²: Media in the Lives of 8- to 18-Year Olds.* Menlo Park, CA: The Henry J. Kaiser Family Foundation; 2010:16.

9 Rideout VJ, Foehr UG, Roberts DF. *Generation M²: Media in the Lives of 8- to 18-Year Olds.* Menlo Park, CA: The Henry J. Kaiser Family Foundation; 2010:9.

10 Rideout VJ, Foehr UG, Roberts DF. *Generation M²: Media in the Lives of 8- to 18-Year Olds.* Menlo Park, CA: The Henry J. Kaiser Family Foundation; 2010:17.

11 Rideout VJ, Foehr UG, Roberts DF. *Generation M²: Media in the Lives of 8- to 18-Year Olds.* Menlo Park, CA: The Henry J. Kaiser Family Foundation; 2010:35.

12 Rideout VJ, Vandewater EA, Wartella EA. *Zero to Six: Electronic Media in the Lives of Infants, Toddlers, and Preschoolers.* Menlo Park, CA: The Henry J. Kaiser Family Foundation; 2003:4.

13 Rideout VJ, Vandewater EA, Wartella EA. *Zero to Six: Electronic Media in the Lives of Infants, Toddlers, and Preschoolers.* Menlo Park, CA: The Henry J. Kaiser Family Foundation; 2003:5.

14 Zimmerman FJ, Christakis DA, Meltzo AN. Television and DVD/video viewing in children younger than 2 years. *Arch Ped Adol Med.* 2007;161:473-479.

15 Rideout VJ, Vandewater EA, Wartella EA. *Zero to Six: Electronic Media in the Lives of Infants, Toddlers, and Preschoolers.* Menlo Park, CA: The Henry J. Kaiser Family Foundation; 2003:4.

16 Rideout VJ, Vandewater EA, Wartella EA. *Zero to Six: Electronic Media in the Lives of Infants, Toddlers, and Preschoolers.* Menlo Park, CA: The Henry J. Kaiser Family Foundation; 2003:11.

17 Rideout VJ, Vandewater EA, Wartella EA. *Zero to Six: Electronic Media in the Lives of Infants, Toddlers, and Preschoolers.* Menlo Park, CA: The Henry J. Kaiser Family Foundation; 2003:6.

18 Rideout VJ, Vandewater EA, Wartella EA. *Zero to Six: Electronic Media in the Lives of Infants, Toddlers, and Preschoolers.* Menlo Park, CA: The Henry J. Kaiser Family Foundation; 2003:4.

19 Rideout VJ, Vandewater EA, Wartella EA. *Zero to Six: Electronic Media in the Lives of Infants, Toddlers, and Preschoolers.* Menlo Park, CA: The Henry J. Kaiser Family Foundation; 2003:7.

20 Rideout VJ, Vandewater EA, Wartella EA. *Zero to Six: Electronic Media in the Lives of Infants, Toddlers, and Preschoolers.* Menlo Park, CA: The Henry J. Kaiser Family Foundation; 2003:7.

21 Crespo CJ, Smit E, Troiano RP, Bartlett SJ, Macera CA, Andersen RE. Television watching, energy intake, and obesity in US children: Results from the Third National Health and Nutrition Examination Survey, 1988-1994. *Arch Pediatr Adolesc Med.* 2001;155:360-365.

22 Janssen I, Katzmarzyk PT, Boyce WF, Vereecken C, Mulvihill, Roberts C, Currie C, Pickett W, and The Health Behaviour in School-Aged Children Obesity Working Group. Comparison of overweight and obesity prevalence in school-aged youth from 34 countries and their relationships with physical activity and dietary patterns. *Obesity Reviews.* 2005;6:123-132.

23 Crespo CJ, Smit E, Troiano RP, Bartlett SJ, Macera CA, Andersen RE. Television watching, energy intake, and obesity in US children: Results from the Third National Health and Nutrition Examination Survey, 1988-1994. *Arch Pediatr Adolesc Med.* 2001;155:360-365.

24 Janssen I, Katzmarzyk PT, Boyce WF, Vereecken C, Mulvihill, Roberts C, Currie C, Pickett W, and The Health Behaviour in School-Aged Children Obesity Working Group. Comparison of overweight and obesity prevalence in school-aged youth from 34 countries and their relationships with physical activity and dietary patterns. *Obesity Reviews.* 2005;6:123-132.

25 Andersen RE, Crespo CJ, Bartlett SJ, Cheskin LJ, Pratt M. Relationship of physical activity and television watching with body weight and level of fatness among children: Results from the Third National Health and Nutrition Examination Survey. *JAMA.* 1998;279:938-942.

26 Crespo CJ, Smit E, Troiano RP, Bartlett SJ, Macera CA, Andersen RE. Television watching, energy intake, and obesity in US children: Results from the Third National Health and Nutrition Examination Survey, 1988-1994. *Arch Pediatr Adolesc Med.* 2001;155:360-365.

27 American Academy of Pediatrics, Committee on Nutrition. Policy Statement: Prevention of pediatric overweight and obesity. *Pediatrics.* 2003;112;424-430.

28 Reilly JJ, Armstrong J, Dorosty AR, Emmett PM, Ness A, Rogers I, Steer C, Sherriff A. Early life risk factors for obesity in childhood: Cohort study. *BMJ.* 2005;330:1357-1359.

29 Lumeng JC, Rahnama S, Appugliese D, Kaciroti N, Bradley RH. Television exposure and overweight risk in preschoolers. *Arch Pediatr Adolesc Med.* 2006;160:417-422.

30 Pagani LS, Fitzpatrick C, Barnett TA, Dubow E. Prospective associations between early childhood television exposure and academic, psychosocial, and physical well-being by middle childhood. *Arch Pediatr Adolesc Med.* 2010;164:425-431.

31 Anderson SE, Whitaker RC. Household routines and obesity in U.S. preschool-aged children. *Pediatrics.* 2010;125:420-428.

32 Lee TH, Ed. Calories burned in 30 minutes for people of three different weights. *Harvard Heart Letter.* Boston, MA: Harvard Health Publications; July 2004. Available at: http://www.health.harvard.edu/newsweek/Calories-burned-in-30-minutes-of-leisure-and-routine-activities.htm. Accessed April 12, 2011.

33 Ebbeling CB, Pawlak DB, Ludwig DS. Childhood obesity: Public-health crisis, common sense cure. *Lancet.* 2002;360:473-482.

34 Hindin TJ, Contento IR, Gussow JD. A media literacy nutrition education curriculum for Head Start parents about the effects of television advertising on their children's food requests. *J Am Diet Assoc.* 2004;104:192-198.

35 Connor SM. Food-related advertising on preschool television: Building brand recognition in young viewers. *Pediatrics.* 2006;118:1478-1485.

36 Chamberlain LJ, Wang Y, Robinson TN. Does children's screen time predict requests for advertised products? Cross-sectional and prospective analyses. *Arch Pediatr Adolesc Med.* 2006;160:363-368.

37 Borzekowski D, Robinson TN. The 30 second effect: An experiment revealing the impact of television commercials on food preferences of preschoolers. *J Am Diet Assoc.* 2001;101:42-46.

38 Weber K, Story M, Harnack L. Internet food marketing strategies aimed at children and adolescents: A content analysis of food and beverage brand web sites. *J Am Diet Assoc.* 2006;106:1463-1466.

39 Alvy LM, Calvert SL. Food marketing on popular children's Web sites: A content analysis. *J Am Diet Assoc.* 2008;108:710-713.

40 Matheson DM, Killen JD, Wang Y, Varady A, Robinson TN. Children's food consumption during television viewing. *Am J Clin Nutr.* 2004;79:1088-1094.

41 Crespo CJ, Smit E, Troiano RP, Bartlett SJ, Macera CA, Andersen RE. Television watching, energy intake, and obesity in US children: Results from the Third National Health and Nutrition Examination Survey, 1988-1994. *Arch Pediatr Adolesc Med.* 2001;155:360-365.

42 Wiecha JL, Peterson KE, Ludwig DS; Kim J, Sobol A, Gortmaker SL. When children eat what they watch: Impact of television viewing on dietary intake in youth. *Arch Pediatr Adolesc Med.* 2006;160:436-442.

43 Francis LA, Birch LL. Does eating during television viewing affect preschool children's intake? *J Am Diet Assoc.* 2006;106:598-600.

44 Francis LA, Birch LL. Does eating during television viewing affect preschool children's intake? *J Am Diet Assoc.* 2006;106:598-600.

45 Wiecha JL, Peterson KE, Ludwig DS; Kim J, Sobol A, Gortmaker SL. When children eat what they watch: Impact of television viewing on dietary intake in youth. *Arch Pediatr Adolesc Med.* 2006;160:436-442.

46 Coon KA, Goldberg J, Rogers BL, Tucker KL. Relationships between use of television during meals and children's food consumption patterns *Pediatrics.* 2001;107:e7. Available at: http://pediatrics.aappublications.org/cgi/content/full/107/1/e7. Accessed April 15, 2010.

47 Robinson, TN. Reducing children's television viewing to prevent obesity: A randomized controlled trial. *JAMA.* 1999;282:1561-1567.

48 Robinson TN. Television viewing and childhood obesity. *Pediatr Clin North Am.* 2001;48:1017-1025.

49 American Academy of Pediatrics, Committee on Public Education. Children, adolescents, and television. *Pediatrics.* 2001;107;423-426.

50 Sharif I, Sargent JD. Association between television, movie, and video game exposure and school performance. *Pediatrics* 2006;118:1061-1070.

51 Waldman M, Nicholson S, Adilov N. *Does Television Cause Autism?* National Bureau of Economic Research; December 2006. Available at http://forum.johnson.cornell.edu/faculty/waldman/autism-waldman-nicholson-adilov.pdf Accessed April 20, 2011.

52 Christakis DA, Zimmerman FJ. Early television exposure and subsequent attentional problems in children. *Pediatrics.* 2004;113:708-713.

53 Zimmerman FJ, Christakis DA, Meltzo AN. Associations between media viewing and language development in children under age 2 years. *J Pediatr.* 2007;151:364-368.

54 Rideout VJ, Vandewater EA, Wartella EA. *Zero to Six: Electronic Media in the Lives of Infants, Toddlers, and Preschoolers.* Menlo Park, CA: The Henry J. Kaiser Family Foundation; 2003:9.

55 Rideout VJ, Foehr UG, Roberts DF. *Generation M²: Media in the Lives of 8- to 18-Year Olds.* Menlo Park, CA: The Henry J. Kaiser Family Foundation; 2010:36.

56 Rideout VJ, Foehr UG, Roberts DF. *Generation M²: Media in the Lives of 8- to 18-Year Olds.* Menlo Park, CA: The Henry J. Kaiser Family Foundation; 2010:4.

57 American Academy of Pediatrics, Committee on Public Education. Children, adolescents, and television. *Pediatrics.* 2001;107;423-426.

58 Sharif I, Sargent JD. Association between television, movie, and video game exposure and school performance. *Pediatrics* 2006;118:1061-1070.

CHAPTER 11: HEALTHY SLEEP, REST, & RELAXATION HABITS

1 Spruyt K, Molfese DL, Gozal D. Sleep duration, sleep regularity, body weight, and metabolic homeostasis in school-aged children. Pediatrics. 2011;127:e345-e352.

2 Lumeng JC, Somashekar D, Appugliese D, Kaciroti N, Corwyn RF, Bradley RH. Shorter sleep duration is associated with increased risk for being overweight at ages 9 to 12 years. *Pediatrics.* 2007;120;1020-1029.

3 Weiss A, Xu F, Storfer-Isser A, Thomas A, Ievers-Landis, Redline S. The association of sleep duration with adolescents' fat and carbohydrate consumption. *Sleep.* 2010;33:1201-1209.

4 Taveras EM, Rifas-Shiman SL, Oken E, Gunderson EP, Gillman, MW. Short sleep duration in infancy and risk of childhood overweight. *Arch Pediatr Adolesc Med.* 2008;162:305-311.

5 Beebe DW, Lewin D, Zeller M, McCabe M, MacLeod K, Daniels SR, Amin R. Sleep in overweight adolescents: shorter sleep, poorer sleep quality, sleepiness, and sleep-disordered breathing. *J Pediatr Psychol.* 2007;32:69-79.

6 Weiss A, Xu F, Storfer-Isser A, Thomas A, Ievers-Landis, Redline S. The association of sleep duration with adolescents' fat and carbohydrate consumption. *Sleep.* 2010;33:1201-1209.

7 Motivala SJ, Irwin MR. Sleep and immunity: Cytokine pathways linking sleep and health outcomes. *Curr Dir Psychol Sci.* 2007;16:21-25.

8 Taheri S. The link between short sleep duration and obesity: We should recommend more sleep to prevent obesity. *Arch Dis Child.* 2006;91:881-884.

9 Taveras EM, Rifas-Shiman SL, Oken E, Gunderson EP, Gillman, MW. Short sleep duration in infancy and risk of childhood overweight. *Arch Pediatr Adolesc Med.* 2008;162:305-311.

10 Snell EK, Adam EK, Duncan GJ. Sleep and the body mass index and overweight status of children and adolescents. *Child Dev.* 2007;78:309-323.

11 Reilly JJ, Armstrong J, Dorosty AR, Emmett PM, Ness A, Rogers I, Steer C, Sherriff A. Early life risk factors for obesity in childhood: Cohort study. *BMJ.* 2005;330:1357-1359.

12 Bell, JF, Zimmerman FJ. Shortened nighttime sleep duration in early life and subsequent childhood obesity. *Arch Pediatr Adolesc Med.* 2010;164:840-845.

13 Anderson SE, Whitaker RC. Household routines and obesity in U.S. preschool-aged children. *Pediatrics.* 2010;125:420-428.

14 Spruyt K, Molfese DL, Gozal D. Sleep duration, sleep regularity, body weight, and metabolic homeostasis in school-aged children. Pediatrics. 2011;127:e345-e352.

15 Bell, JF, Zimmerman FJ. Shortened nighttime sleep duration in early life and subsequent childhood obesity. *Arch Pediatr Adolesc Med.* 2010;164:840-845.

16 Weiss A, Xu F, Storfer-Isser A, Thomas A, Ievers-Landis, Redline S. The association of sleep duration with adolescents' fat and carbohydrate consumption. *Sleep.* 2010;33:1201-1209.

17 Taheri S. The link between short sleep duration and obesity: We should recommend more sleep to prevent obesity. *Arch Dis Child.* 2006;91:881-884.

18 Taheri S. The link between short sleep duration and obesity: We should recommend more sleep to prevent obesity. *Arch Dis Child.* 2006;91:881-884.

19 Lumeng JC, Somashekar D, Appugliese D, Kaciroti N, Corwyn RF, Bradley RH. Shorter sleep duration is associated with increased risk for being overweight at ages 9 to 12 years. *Pediatrics.* 2007;120;1020-1029.

20 Beebe DW, Lewin D, Zeller M, McCabe M, MacLeod K, Daniels SR, Amin R. Sleep in overweight adolescents: shorter sleep, poorer sleep quality, sleepiness, and sleep-disordered breathing. *J Pediatr Psychol.* 2007;32:69-79.

21 Gupta NK, Mueller WH, Chan W, Meininger JC. Is obesity associated with poor sleep quality in adolescents? *Am J Hum Biol.* 2002;14:762-768.

22 Chen MY, Wang EK, Jeng YJ. Adequate sleep among adolescents is positively associated with health status and health-related behaviors. *BMC Public Health.* 2006;6:59.

23 Weiss A, Xu F, Storfer-Isser A, Thomas A, Ievers-Landis, Redline S. The association of sleep duration with adolescents' fat and carbohydrate consumption. *Sleep.* 2010;33:1201-1209.

24 Beebe DW, Lewin D, Zeller M, McCabe M, MacLeod K, Daniels SR, Amin R. Sleep in overweight adolescents: shorter sleep, poorer sleep quality, sleepiness, and sleep-disordered breathing. *J Pediatr Psychol.* 2007;32:69-79.

25 Sung V, Harriet Hiscock H, Sciberras E, Efron D. Sleep problems in children with attention-deficit/hyperactivity disorder: Prevalence and the effect on the child and family. *Arch Pediatr Adolesc Med.* 2008;162:336-342.

26 Sung V, Harriet Hiscock H, Sciberras E, Efron D. Sleep problems in children with attention-deficit/hyperactivity disorder: Prevalence and the effect on the child and family. *Arch Pediatr Adolesc Med.* 2008;162:336-342.

27 Owens JA, Maxim R, Nobile C, McGuinn M, Msall M. Parental and self-report of sleep in children with attention-deficit/hyperactivity disorder. *Arch Pediatr Adolesc Med.* 2000;154:549-555.

28 Millman RP, Working Group on Sleepiness in Adolescents/Young Adults, AAP Committee on Adolescence. Excessive sleepiness in adolescents and young adults: Causes, consequences, and treatment strategies. *Pediatrics.* 2005;115;1774-1786.

29 Millman RP, Working Group on Sleepiness in Adolescents/Young Adults, AAP Committee on Adolescence. Excessive sleepiness in adolescents and young adults: Causes, consequences, and treatment strategies. *Pediatrics.* 2005;115;1774-1786.

30 Sung V, Harriet Hiscock H, Sciberras E, Efron D. Sleep problems in children with attention-deficit/hyperactivity disorder: Prevalence and the effect on the child and family. *Arch Pediatr Adolesc Med.* 2008;162:336-342.

31 Millman RP, Working Group on Sleepiness in Adolescents/Young Adults, AAP Committee on Adolescence. Excessive sleepiness in adolescents and young adults: Causes, consequences, and treatment strategies. *Pediatrics.* 2005;115;1774-1786.

32 Millman RP, Working Group on Sleepiness in Adolescents/Young Adults, AAP Committee on Adolescence. Excessive sleepiness in adolescents and young adults: Causes, consequences, and treatment strategies. *Pediatrics.* 2005;115;1774-1786.

33 National Sleep Foundation. *Children and Sleep.* Available at: http://www.sleepfoundation.org/article/sleep-topics/children-and-sleep. Accessed June 28, 2011.

34 National Sleep Foundation. *Children and Sleep.* Available at: http://www.sleepfoundation.org/article/sleep-topics/children-and-sleep. Accessed June 28, 2011.

35 National Sleep Foundation. *Teens and Sleep.* Available at: http://www.sleepfoundation.org/article/sleep-topics/teens-and-sleep. Accessed June 28, 2011.

36 Millman RP, Working Group on Sleepiness in Adolescents/Young Adults, AAP Committee on Adolescence. Excessive sleepiness in adolescents and young adults: Causes, consequences, and treatment strategies. *Pediatrics.* 2005;115;1774-1786.

37 National Sleep Foundation. *Women and Sleep.* Available at: http://www.sleepfoundation.org/article/sleep-topics/women-and-sleep. Accessed June 28, 2011.

38 Taheri S. The link between short sleep duration and obesity: We should recommend more sleep to prevent obesity. *Arch Dis Child.* 2006;91:881-884.

39 Edens G. Sleep tight: Healthy sleep for the whole family. *ParentLife.* May 2010;16:40.

40 Edens G. Sleep tight: Healthy sleep for the whole family. *ParentLife.* May 2010;16:40.

41 Taheri S. The link between short sleep duration and obesity: We should recommend more sleep to prevent obesity. *Arch Dis Child.* 2006;91:881-884.

42 Taheri S. The link between short sleep duration and obesity: We should recommend more sleep to prevent obesity. *Arch Dis Child.* 2006;91:881-884.

43 Millman RP, Working Group on Sleepiness in Adolescents/Young Adults, AAP Committee on Adolescence. Excessive sleepiness in adolescents and young adults: Causes, consequences, and treatment strategies. *Pediatrics.* 2005;115;1774-1786.

44 Peeke PM, Chrousos GP. Hypercortisolism and obesity. *Ann NY Acad Sci.* 1995;771:665-676.

45 Epel ES, McEwen B, Seeman T, Matthews K, Castellazzo G, Brownell KD, Bell J, Ickovics JR. Stress and body shape: stress-induced cortisol secretion is consistently greater among women with central fat. *Psychosom Med.* 2000; 62:623-632.

46 Epel E, Lapidus R, McEwen B, Brownell K. Stress may add bite to appetite in women: A laboratory study of stress-induced cortisol and eating behavior. *Psychoneuroendocrinology.* 2001;26:37-49.

47 Archer R. *The Leadership Lock: Nine Keys to Free the Leader Within You.* Puyallup, WA: Lifeline Publishing; 2004:107. Reprinted by Permission of Roger Archer.

48 Twenge JM, Gentile B, DeWall CN, Ma D, Lacefield K, Schurtz DR. Birth cohort increases in psychopathology among young Americans, 1938–2007: A cross-temporal meta-analysis of the MMPI. *Clin Psychol Rev.* 2010;30:145-154.

49 Archer R. *The Leadership Lock: Nine Keys to Free the Leader Within You.* Puyallup, WA: Lifeline Publishing; 2004:89. Reprinted by Permission of Roger Archer.

50 Morgan E, Kuykendall C. *What Every Child Needs: Meet Your Child's Nine Basic Needs for Love.* Grand Rapids, MI: Zondervan; 1997:185. Reprinted by Permission of MOPS International.

CHAPTER 12: A BYPRODUCT OF OUR CULTURE

1 Wang Y, Lobstein T. Worldwide trends in childhood overweight and obesity. *International Journal of Pediatric Obesity.* 2006;1:11-25.

2 Ogden CL, Carroll MD, Curtin LR, McDowell MA, Tabak CJ, Flegal KM. Prevalence of overweight and obesity in the United States, 1999-2004. *JAMA.* 2006;295:1549-1555.

3 Wang Y, Lobstein T. Worldwide trends in childhood overweight and obesity. *International Journal of Pediatric Obesity*. 2006;1:11-25.

4 World Health Organization, Media Centre. *Obesity and overweight, Fact Sheet No. 311*. Updated March 2011. Available at http://www.who.int/mediacentre/factsheets/fs311/en/index.html. Accessed October 3, 2011.

5 Wang Y, Lobstein T. Worldwide trends in childhood overweight and obesity. *International Journal of Pediatric Obesity*. 2006;1:11-25.

6 Janssen I, Katzmarzyk PT, Boyce WF, Vereecken C, Mulvihill C, Roberts C, Currie C, Pickett W. Comparison of overweight and obesity prevalence in school-aged youth from 34 countries and their relationships with physical activity and dietary patterns. *Obesity Reviews*. 2005;6:123-132.

7 Lobstein T, Baur L, Uauy R. Obesity in children and young people: A crisis in public health. *Obesity Reviews*. 2004;5:4-85.

8 International Obesity Taskforce. *The Global Epidemic*. Available at: http://www.iaso.org/iotf/obesity/obesitytheglobalepidemic/. Accessed October 3, 2011.

9 International Obesity Taskforce. *The Global Epidemic*. Available at: http://www.iaso.org/iotf/obesity/obesitytheglobalepidemic/. Accessed October 3, 2011.

10 World Health Organization, Media Centre. *Obesity and overweight, Fact Sheet No. 311*. Updated March 2011. Available at http://www.who.int/mediacentre/factsheets/fs311/en/index.html. Accessed October 3, 2011.

11 Wang Y, Lobstein T. Worldwide trends in childhood overweight and obesity. *International Journal of Pediatric Obesity*. 2006;1:11-25.

12 *FAQ's*. McDonald's Canada. Available at: http://www.mcdonalds.ca/en/aboutus/faq.aspx. Accessed October 4, 2010

13 Wiecha JL, Finkelstein D, Troped PJ, Fragala M, Peterson KE. School vending machine use and fast-food restaurant use are associated with sugar-sweetened beverage intake in youth. *J Am Diet Assoc*. 2006;106:1624-1630.

14 Li Y, Hu X, Zhang Q, Liu A, Fang H, Hao L, Duan Y, Xu H, Shang X, Ma J, Xu G, Du L, Li Y, Guo H, Li T, Ma G. The nutrition-based comprehensive intervention study on childhood obesity in China (NISCOC): A randomised cluster controlled trial. *BMC Public Health*. 2010;10:229.

15 Wang Y, Mi J, Shan XY, Wang QJ, Ge KY. Is China facing an obesity epidemic and the consequences? The trends in obesity and chronic disease in China. *Int J Obes*. 2007;31:177-188.

16 Wu Y. Overweight and obesity in China: The once lean giant has a weight problem that is increasing rapidly. *BMJ*. 2006;333:362–363.

17 Wu Y. Overweight and obesity in China: The once lean giant has a weight problem that is increasing rapidly. *BMJ*. 2006;333:362–363.

18 Wang Y, Mi J, Shan XY, Wang QJ, Ge KY. Is China facing an obesity epidemic and the consequences? The trends in obesity and chronic disease in China. *Int J Obes*. 2007;31:177-188.

19 Popkin BM. Will China's nutrition transition overwhelm its health care system and slow economic growth? *Health Aff*. 2008;27:1064-1076.

20 Li Y, Hu X, Zhang Q, Liu A, Fang H, Hao L, Duan Y, Xu H, Shang X, Ma J, Xu G, Du L, Li Y, Guo H, Li T, Ma G. The nutrition-based comprehensive intervention study on childhood obesity in China (NISCOC): A randomised cluster controlled trial. *BMC Public Health.* 2010;10:229.

21Wang Y, Mi J, Shan XY, Wang QJ, Ge KY. Is China facing an obesity epidemic and the consequences? The trends in obesity and chronic disease in China. *Int J Obes.* 2007;31:177-188.

22 Popkin BM. Will China's nutrition transition overwhelm its health care system and slow economic growth? *Health Aff.* 2008;27:1064-1076.

23 Wu Y. Overweight and obesity in China: The once lean giant has a weight problem that is increasing rapidly. *BMJ.* 2006;333:362–363.

24 Levine JA. Obesity in China: Causes and solutions. *Chinese Medical Journal.* 2007;120:1043- 1050.

25 Archer R. *The Leadership Lock: Nine Keys to Free the Leader Within You.* Puyallup, WA: Lifeline Publishing; 2004:157. Reprinted by Permission of Roger Archer.

26 Sammons MB. Moms and drinking: Secret after-hour addictions of working mothers. *ParentDish.* October 27, 2010. Available at: http://www.parentdish.com/2010/10/27/moms-and-drinking. Accessed September 8, 2011.

27 DeGregory L. Addicted moms: Everybody knows somebody. *Working Mother.* October 2010. Available at: http://www.workingmother.com/special-reports/addicted-moms-everybody-knows-somebody. Accessed September 8, 2011.

28 Reisser P. From the experts: From Dr. Paul Reisser. *Focus on the Family Magazine.* November 2006;30:29. Reprinted by Permission of Dr. Paul Reisser.

29 Reisser P. From the experts: From Dr. Paul Reisser. *Focus on the Family Magazine.* November 2006;30:29. Reprinted by Permission of Dr. Paul Reisser.

About the Author

A Registered Dietitian (RD) for over ten years, Keeley has practiced in a variety of settings: long-term care and rehabilitation; public health and community nutrition; and outpatient nutrition counseling and education. Keeley's specialties include pediatric nutrition, weight management, maternal nutrition and lactation, food allergies and intolerances, and cardiovascular disease.

Keeley graduated *Summa Cum Laude* from Seattle Pacific University with a Bachelor of Science in Food and Nutrition and a Dietetics Specialization. She went on to complete her dietetic internship at Baylor University Medical Center in Dallas, where she received the Distinguished Dietetic Intern Award and Scholarship.

Keeley began her writing career as a contributing writer for a nutrition website, HealthCastle.com. She has also had articles published by various magazines and websites as well as cited on sites such as LiveStrong.com and eHow.com. Please visit Keeley's websites at PoisoiningOurChildren.com and TGBGnutrition.com.

Made in the USA
Lexington, KY
25 October 2013